Consciousness of Health:
Tuning-In To Absolute Well-Being

Kidest OM ॐ

CONSCIOUSNESS OF HEALTH:
TUNING IN TO ABSOLUTE WELL-BEING
by Kidest OM ॐ
Copyright © 2011

Contents

Introduction

Section I: A Shift in Paradigm – Upgrading Your Consciousness Operating System
- I   Redefining Your Belief Boundaries
- II   You Are A Conscious Energy Being
- III   Your Emotional Indicators
- IV   Faulty Programs Formed On The Premise of Resistance
- V   Your Multidimensional Reality Platform
- VI   Shifting To A New Frequency Domain
- VII   Redefining Disease

Section II: Daily Exercises
- VIII   The Power of Practice
- IX   Body Scan
- X   Energy Work
- XI   Contemplation
- XII   Presence
- XIII   Positive Focus
- XIV   Appreciate
- XV   Daily Release

Section III: The Workbook
- Instructions
- Suggested Guidelines
- Stream 1 to 40

- XVI   There Is Only Consciousness
- XVII   Your Power To Choose
- XVIII Declaration of Intrinsic Power

"Every human being is the author of his own health or disease."

— Siddhartha Gautama, The Buddha

SECTION I
A SHIFT IN PARADIGM – UPGRADING YOUR CONSCIOUSNESS OPERATING SYSTEM

Introduction

The key premises of this book are:
- *Consciousness is the sole cause and source of your manifested experience.*

- *You are Consciousness.*

- *You live in a space-time platform composed purely of energy and empty space.*

- *Your physical health is a manifestation of your consciousness, there are no other factors.*

- *Your experience of your physical health can shift in proportion to your shift in consciousness.*

- *You **can** change your materialized body-Universe reality naturally by changing your vibration, by allowing an energetic shift in consciousness, by allowing a change in the frequency field that you are.*

Inquiry and study directed at the world of form, of manifested outcomes, conditions, and circumstances will not provide an ultimate answer or solution to the problems experienced in your waking world. The manifested world and all that it contains is a secondary reality, so at best, all it can offer are temporary overlays that will mask the problems already present. Albert Einstein is often quoted as saying that you cannot solve a problem with the same consciousness that brought forth the problem in the first place. In this same way, you cannot experience improved realities while still remaining in the consciousness that brought forth the reality you currently appear to be experiencing. It is consciousness that is at cause of all that appears. It is consciousness that is the source of the waking world you participate in. Circumstances, conditions, manifestations in the world of form are meaningless and powerless for they are only effects, they are only shadows, they are only reflections. To look to the manifested world for answers and explanations is to look at your shadow with the hopes of knowing your name. Shadows are lifeless reflections. They hold no answers. The only level of experience which will allow for total change in what appears, is a change in consciousness itself. It is only at the level of cause that you can bring about any true and lasting transformation.

Every perspective you hold, every psychological standpoint in your mental possession propels you into a unique Universe of experience with its own set of rules. The way in which you conceive of your world and yourself places you into a body-Universe reality that will mirror, reflect, and validate your conceptions. Your Universe will not contradict you for you and your Universe are intimately unified. And so it is only when you begin to transform your internal psyche, your attitudes, your beliefs, your very model of reality that the Universe and the rules within which you play transform as well. This is about impelling a shift in consciousness, it is always about inducing a shift in your own internal structure – the lens and frequency from which you experience your world. It is the alteration of your own consciousness that allows you to alter every dimension of your physical experience.

As the human organism moves into a new realm

of experience, old systems dissolve to make room for a worldview that is more in line with a more expanded dimension of being. Humanity is on the whole awakening into an expanded perspective, a higher frequency platform and dimension that allows for immediate change and instant transformation. More and more beings are beginning to shed old models of limitation and materialism based attitudes in favor of the experience of a vibrational reality, a universe of energy in constant motion, a life of malleable circumstances and outcomes. The stream of consciousness offered in this book is designed to serve as a bridge into that shift by calling you to stretch your ideas, your definitions, and your expectations around your physical experience. It is by your capacity to contemplate ideas vibrating at different frequencies that you allow yourself to participate in different realties. The faster the spin of the ideas you hold in yourself, the more malleable the world you encounter in waking consciousness.

Every model has its limitation. Every system of thought is by its nature a conditioning of the Infinite Unknown. And yet each system of thought, each model of reality you hold introduces you to a unique energetic platform from which to observe and participate in your world. New definitions lead to new experiences, and this book offers that. It offers a new way to look at everything you take to be your world, your body, your Universe so that you can experience the true power inherent in who and what you really are. It is in your ability to change your ideas of self and the world that you live and experience the power of your being.

You cannot hold a limited view of yourself and

this space-time platform, you cannot define yourself and your world as fixed and unchanging, and access the limitless possibilities that permeate your world and your own being. It is by changing the consciousness with which you experience your world that you allow the structure and appearance of your reality to change.

— Kidest OM

I.   REDEFINING YOUR BELIEF BOUNDARIES

As the course of your physical embodiment unfolds, you have picked up innumerable beliefs about who you are and what your world is. You have beliefs about your reality. You have well rehearsed stories about who you are. You have beliefs about your physical body, what it is, what it can or cannot do. You have beliefs about health. You have beliefs about the absence of health. You have awareness of names upon names of maladies, symptoms, illnesses and diseases that you believe determine your well-being. You have accumulated countless stories and endless evidence for the existence of sickness. And for the most part, you have assumed the perspective that the state of your physical health and well-being is in the hands of factors outside of you.

Your physical Universe however does not assert any conditions upon you. The interconnected matrix of your experience does not impose circumstances and conditions upon you. There are no forced experiences or uninvited conditions. There are no random symptoms or accidental illnesses. Whether you are consciously aware of it or not, you ask for and so observe into being every experience that manifests in and as your body-Universe reality. You are the creator of your personal reality, and your physical system, your physical body is one of the many aspects of your experience that obeys the boundaries you have erected.

The Unified Field in which you exist supports you unconditionally in the reality you create through the beliefs you have embedded in your outlook and through the numberless programs you install into your consciousness-matrix. Stay with this thought for a moment – every possible disease or symptom known to you is a program you have installed into your consciousness-matrix. In effect, you have taught your physical system to play out programs, patterns of information, so that you can experience the diseases, illnesses, and symptoms you believe are a part of being human.

You are so powerful that whatever you accept as valid information, as a valid virus or any other cause of disease, in your time-space reality, manifests in your experience. What you know to be true, appears. What you know to be real, the beliefs you have rehearsed silently within yourself make themselves known to you as your physical body and personal reality. And so, it is in the identifying and changing of these beliefs, in the expansion of the ideas you have up to now formed, that your day to day experience of physicality can shift to look and feel as you now consciously choose for them to look and feel. It is up to you to un-install these programs. It is up to you to see through the illusion of the manifested world and into the causal role of the consciousness that you are.

You are not at the mercy of factors outside of you. You have never been at the mercy of seemingly external factors. There are no authorities greater than you in your own personal reality. You are one hundred percent responsible for the body-Universe reality you tune into and experience as your physical world. You are the sole author of all that you make manifest in and as your experience.

In the moment you return the power of causality back to your own consciousness, in the instant you let your own consciousness be the sole cause of all that you experience, you return the power to change and transform your world back to yourself. Are you ready to do that now? Are you now willing to be the sole author of all that you experience? Are you ready to unknow what you have up to now believed about what your body is and the level of well-being you are capable of experiencing in this reality?

II.   YOU ARE A CONSCIOUS ENERGY BEING

Every aspect of the human experience is a translation of energy patterns. Your body-brain system is constantly converting unique wave patterns into the sensory world you appear to experience moment after moment. What you experience as touch is a translation of vibrational data. What you experience as taste, smell, sight, what you experience as any and all sensation is the registration of electrical data, of information, by your nervous system that is then reconstructed as a three dimensional "something" by your brain. What you experience as thought, is a registration of energy. Everything you experience as the physical body, the brain, the heart, every organ, cell, and bone is itself a translation of a unique frequency field. *Take yourself to each body part and allow yourself to recognize it as a pattern of light and information. Allow yourself to experience every organ, every extremity, and every sensory system, every single one of your trillions of cells, as pure light. Let yourself feel what it feels like to see and experience these "body" parts as frequency fields, as a network of particles dispersed in empty space.*

Each and every attribute of the world you right now perceive as physical is a three-dimensional representation of wave patterns, electric signals recorded by the body-brain system. You do not experience a solid physical world. No actual physical world exists as you have traditionally believed there to exist. No actual physical body exists as you have traditionally believed to exist. The fixed physical environment you appear to experience, the seemingly solid body that appears as your own, is in fact the convincing illusion created by the relationship between the continuously fluctuating energy field, and your translating body-brain system. You recurrently experience unique translations of vibration that your brain-body system reconstructs as a physical reality. It is energetic pulsations that appear to you as your physical material environment.

So what is the true nature of your being that everything about your world is a reconstruction of electrical data? What is it about your being that you only understand a world of electrical signals, of vibrational information?

You are a being of Light. You are electrical, you are energy. Everything about you, all the octaves of your being, is energy. You are photons and information. You are Light patterning in specific ways in accord to the ideas you hold about who you are and what your world is. You are wave-patterns and empty space. You are pure Consciousness, an intricate intelligent energy system. And it is learning to experience your reality from this dimension of perception that will allow you to experience the malleability of everything you take to be a physical reality.

Every idea you entertain is vibrating at a specific frequency and so has its own vibrational density. The vibrational density of your perception determines how and in what ways you experience physical reality. The higher the frequencies of your self-definitions, the higher the frequencies of the ideas you encode into your consciousness-matrix, the more flexible and fluid your experience of physical reality.

The paradigm of physicality, of fixed and unchanging material substance, is of its own vibrational density and births its own set of experiences – it births its own unique vibrational platform, or in familiar words, it is its own unique world. All that determines how you experience your body-Universe reality is the line up of ideas, the vibrational lens, through which you look out onto your preferred body-Universe reality. It is entirely within your power to choose what perceptual field, what vibrational density or domain you will experience your body-Universe reality through.

You are not a material being. You are not a physical being. You are not solid matter. There is no such thing as solid matter. What appears as solid matter is predominately empty space with highly vibrating particles dispersed through it. Physicality is an illusion you engage in moment after moment. Physicality is a shared hallucination you participate in frame after frame. You are an energy being. You are all Light. You are all Consciousness. You are a field of vibrational patterns. Your physical body is energy vibrating at a specific frequency. What you take to be cells and muscle tissue, bones and organs, are all composed of particles in constant motion. Every emotion you experience is energy vibrating at specific frequencies. Your thoughts are energies vibrating at a specific frequency. Every octave of your being, every level of your multidimensional being, is energy. And your beliefs, your practiced pattern of thinking and the line-up of ideas you have rehearsed in this reality up to now, make up your dominant vibrational state of being.

What kind of body-Universe reality you experience is completely dependent upon your dominant vibrational state of being. In an energetic reality view, you see all things as patterns of light and information. You view all that appears on your screen of experience as particles in movement flickering in and out of numberless positions. All appears in constant motion, all appears in constant flux. This is a significantly different angle of view than a view of the world as material, as fixed. In your recognition that you are not a physical body in a physical room or environment, that you are a vibrational being in a vibrational environment, you give yourself access to a different set of probabilities to actualize into your experience. One view presents you with a body-Universe that you have to chisel and hammer into shape, that you have to physically alter into your vision of well-being, while the other offers you a much more fluid and malleable body-Universe where a subtle shift in consciousness translates as a physical shift in the body-Universe. Regardless of which body-Universe reality you choose to participate in and attune yourself to, the common denominator is you.

What determines the body-Universe reality you experience is you, your own beliefs, your own ideas, what you are conscious of being. Upgrading your self-identity to that of an "energy being" rather than a "physical being" brings with it its own set of experiences. Dwell frequently in this vibrational domain – the domain of knowing yourself to be all energy all the time. Let yourself marinate in this new arena of experience. The moment you begin to shift your definitions, who and what you take yourself to be, is the moment you move yourself into a different vibrational domain, a different Universe with its own set of parameters. You do not experience anything in your reality as it truly is, you experience only what you take yourself to be. You experience only the self-definitions and ideas you have about your world. Nothing in this Universe is fixed, nothing simply "is". You take probabilities from the Unified Field of infinite potential and you actualize them into being based on your ideas of your world and yourself. You and how you perceive yourself and your world are *that* powerful.

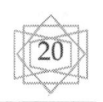

III. YOUR EMOTIONAL INDICATORS

Emotions are not arbitrary or random experiences of being a (seemingly) physical human. The mathematical precision of this space-time platform is methodical in every layer of its creation. Everything has a useful purpose. You are receiving constant communication and tangible immediate feedback on how pure energy, the universal power that animates your entire existence and world, is flowing through your physical apparatus. Your physical system is perfectly designed to indicate to you how energy is flowing through it in any given moment so that you are aware of your own vitality and optimal functioning. Emotions, what you translate as an emotional experience, are an experience of this guidance of energy flow. Emotions are guidance; they are a tangible experiential feedback on the availability of power within your physical vehicle. Just like most of your digital devices offer you a reading of available power, battery readings informing you when you need to re-charge or re-connect to a power-source, your emotions offer you a similar type of reading.

What you experience as positive emotions are indicating to you that you are freely allowing the flow of life energy through your physical system. In the states you translate as happy, joyful, appreciative, or any other "high" feeling state, you are receiving communication that you are fully charged and connected to Universal power. Make note of the language you use in these instances – uplifted, full, light, high – all of these are words that point to you of what is happening in your positive states of experience.

What you experience as negative emotions are indicating to you that you are disallowing the flow of life energy through your physical system. In these instances, for whatever reason, universal power is not being allowed to flow freely through all your numberless energy meridians. Negative emotions are indicating to you that you are running on low, that your power supply is low. And again the language you use in these instances indicates to you what is happening in your physical system. In negative states, you often use words like "I feel low" or "I feel down" which is exactly what is happening in the physical apparatus. In the negative states you translate as anger, frustration, confusion, or depression, there is a much lower flow of Universal power, and your overall power supply is down, has decreased. All that you experience as an emotion in any given moment, is indicating to you the degree to which you are allowing or disallowing the flow of life energy, the flow of Universal power, what you've called in various traditions as Prana, Chi, Tao, Rei, Mana throughout your history, to flow through your physical apparatus. Emotions are communication. Emotions are guidance. Emotions are indicators of energy flow. Emotions are feedback on the availability of power throughout the physical system, the physical vehicle you experience as your body.

    The thoughts that you think and all that you focus on in your waking world act as the valves that open or constrict the energy channels or meridians of your physical apparatus. The better you feel, the more positive points of focus that you hold, the more pure energy you are receiving and flowing through your physical system. The better you feel, the higher the vibrations or frequencies you attune yourself to. The energies that you translate as joy, love, appreciation, excitement, certainty, are all indicating to you that your vibration is "high", that all your energy channels are open and life energy, or universal power, is moving through your system freely and without restriction. That you are tuned in, plugged in, tapped in fully to the flow of Universal power. While your negative emotions are telling you that because of your chosen point of focus, because of the thoughts you are focusing on within yourself, you are tuned out, tapped out, unplugged from the flow of Universal power. Now although you never fully unplug, although there is a layer of your multidimensional being that is always plugged in because you cannot at all operate or function in the world of waking consciousness without Universal power, what this description is pointing out to you is that you do either enhance or diminish the overall flow of this Universal power, and you have the built-in guidance system to let you know exactly what you are doing as you focus on specific thought-streams.

Energy is the language of the Universe. Everything physical and non-physical is in a constant vibrational dialogue. Vibration is your non-physical language of communication with everything visible and invisible to you in your world. Not only are you a vibrational transmitter and receiver constantly and continuously projecting a specific, unique signal, but you are an entirely vibrational being through and through. You are at all times pure Light and information encoding your body-matrix with the frequencies you stay tuned into. Everything in the

Universe responds predominately to your energetic broadcast, your dominant vibrational output, or your unique vibrational signature. Your first language is not words, but the frequency broadcast of your own being. Your primary language is energy, the basic substance of all that you experience. And this is why you can pick up on the "vibes" of one another without ever needing words. You pick up on the states of other beings and the energetic state of a room you walk in, because your whole world and everything in it is all vibration.

    What you communicate, just as what you create, and how energy flows through your physical apparatus is entirely within your power. You have absolute control over what your personal vibration is, what your frequency-of-being is. You have control over what you vibrate. You have control over what you broadcast. You have control over what you dominantly emanate and radiate out into your environment. You have control over how much universal power you allow to flow through you because you are given constant feedback. Your emotions are telling you exactly how much universal power you are allowing yourself to flow. This gives you a chance to redirect your focus anytime you are pinching off the flow through your points of focus. This feedback system gives you access to immediate guidance on fuel or power availability so that you can tune in, tap in, plug in whenever you seem to be going off course. There is no need to create stories around the emotions being experienced. Simply recognizing them as energy flow indicators and making the course correction necessary is all that is required. You have absolute authority over your personal vibration and the energetic environment you create through your physical body, your unique physical system of creation.

You are the sole author of the body-Universe reality you materialize and participate in.

IV. FAULTY PROGRAMS FORMED ON THE PREMISE OF RESISTANCE

There is only absolute well-being or your learned resistance to it. Absolute well-being pervades all of existence. Well-being, perfection in every way, is the foundational nature of the power that manifests as your physical Universe and everything within it. In your physical experience, premises have been formed from the perspective of resistance. Resistance only means the disallowing of well-being, the closing off to it, and the forming of beliefs in something other than well-being.

When you hold that absolute well-being is not possible, you are resisting well-being. When you hold that dis-ease is a natural and normal occurrence of being a physical human, you are resisting well-being. It is only from a state of resistance that ideas of disease and illness have been normalized and accepted to be part of physical experience. Absolute well-being is the only norm, as absolute well-being is the core principle of the Universe.

Let go of the belief that disease is natural. Let go of the belief that symptoms are common experiences. Let go of the belief that it is natural for the body to experience anything other than continued absolute well-being. What if there are human beings all over your world that never experience disease? Are you open to the possibility that such a thing exists? It does.

Examples of faulty programs:

∞ *Disease is natural.*

- ∞ Sickness and illness are natural parts of physical experience.
- ∞ It's normal to get sick.
- ∞ Everybody gets sick.
- ∞ Everybody gets the flu.
- ∞ Everybody gets old.
- ∞ Sickness is just a part of life.
- ∞ Physical decline is natural.
- ∞ Physical degeneration is natural.
- ∞ Everybody experiences breakdown as they age.
- ∞ Recovery takes time.
- ∞ Healing takes time.
- ∞ The body doesn't know how to come back into balance.
- ∞ I only have one option.
- ∞ Diagnoses are real and true.
- ∞ Diagnoses are final.
- ∞ Symptoms mean sickness is inevitable.
- ∞ I can get sick.
- ∞ I have to fight my sickness.
- ∞ I'm vulnerable and susceptible to what the world says is happening.
- ∞ My well-being is in the hands of things outside of me.
- ∞ Things outside of me decide the fate of my physical health.
- ∞ What other beings have manifested into their physical system applies to me.
- ∞ Someone else's indicator of resistance applies to me.
- ∞ If I focus and complain about the discord in my body, it will go away.
- ∞ The path to my well-being is physical action.
- ∞ It is something external that makes me experience physical disease.

- ∞ What the world tells me is real applies to me.
- ∞ I am at the mercy of world definitions.
- ∞ I have to tell my body how to behave.
- ∞ My body is a clump of flesh and bones.
- ∞ I know more about my body's well-being than my body does.
- ∞ There are outside experts of my physical body.

The faulty programs you have accumulated and have made natural are many, and as you learn to experience physical reality from a different vibrational density, through a more expanded lens of being an energetic being in an energetic world, these false premises will make themselves known and visible to you. As they do, you can easily dissolve your entanglement with them. You can simply un-install them from the field of consciousness that you are, from your consciousness-matrix.

Whatever information you integrate into yourself, into the consciousness that you are, can be released anytime at your choosing. No belief is permanent. You are not stuck with or destined to live out your human experience attached to belief programs that no longer work for you or serve you. As you wake up to the various programs you have accepted and installed into your reality-matrix, you also wake up to your power to experience something different.

So what are you ready to let go of?
What limiting false premise are you now ready to release?

V. YOUR MULTIDIMENSIONAL REALITY PLATFORM & SELF

You are a multi-dimensional consciousness experiencing the nature of physical focus. You are a multi-octave being simultaneously existing in numerous worlds. Consciousness is not an isolated stream. It is a stream that branches and flows in countless directions, into countless possibilities, into innumerable realities. You are this same consciousness. You are this infinite stream of well-being. You are not a limited being having to beat a desired reality into manifestation. You are not a limited fixed occurrence in the ocean of existence. You are all possible waves on the ocean's surface. You are already all possibilities in Creation.

You are not your body, nor are you your mind. Scan your physical system and try and locate yourself. Are you the hands, the feet, or the ears? In which set of cells or single cell do you reside? Where are you located in the body? And if you are located in the body, how are you able to become aware of the inside or the outside of the body? If you were to place the body on an operating table, where would you be found?

You are prior to the body-mind dimension of being that emerges as you enter your waking world. Your physical system is a highly complex vehicle designed to allow you to navigate in your own unique translation of this space-time platform. It is an extension of you, but it is not all of you. Your day to day conscious mind is an intelligent extension designed to allow you to bring into focus realities you have chosen to experience. Yet again, this too is not all that you are.

What you experience as your body-mind system in the waking world is a necessary conception of this space-time platform; it is this sensory-system that allows you to experience a physical world full of physical events. It is your interface to earth-reality. But you are more than this body-mind interface.

The more you begin to recognize yourself as a field of consciousness, the more you expand your identity to include more than the vehicles of consciousness that you experience as a body and mind, the more you allow your true boundless form to emerge. And it is from this unbounded sense of being that you will experience the power inherent in who and what you really are. It is when you recognize your vehicles as vehicles that you can effectively utilize them to bring about the experiences you desire.

The Unified Source Field in which you have your being and move within has numberless worlds, countless potential realities vibrating ready to be accessed and experienced by you. And the infinite frequencies of all of Creation share but One space – the space in which you right now appear to be. Every one of these worlds, every potential reality has within in it a matching version of the you that you take yourself to be, the interference pattern that you experience as yourself frame after frame. All of creation already contains within it all possibilities. The space in which you right now appear to be already contains within it an infinite number of alternate realities. Nothing is incomplete. Nothing has yet to be formed. Nothing has yet to be created or finished. It is all already done. It is all a living reality in this moment. All potentialities, all possibilities, are already living realities in the Unified

Source Field you are right now within.

That you exist in a Unified Field of Infinite Possibility is an ever-emerging stream of understanding making itself known in your current space-time platform. In your powerful and eternal Now exist all possibilities, all outcomes, and all possible versions of your own unique pattern of self.

There is already a vibrant and lively you in this powerful instant. There is already a reality in existence right now in which you are an expression of absolute well-being in all forms. And it is the signal, the vibrational tone, of this unique you that you shift in to as you mobilize and actualize a shift in consciousness.

Your power rests in your ability to vibrate at and attune your focus to the frequency domain, the unique vibrational density, of your preferred stream of experience. This responsive and interactive space-time platform that you experience as your physical body-Universe reality is ever sensitive and immediate to the shifts in frequency you generate within yourself, within the vibrational field of consciousness that you are.

You are the sole author, definer, and perceiver of all that you make manifest in and as your personal physical reality.

VI. SHIFTING TO A NEW FREQUENCY DOMAIN

Living your physical experience with the expansive perspective of being an energetic being in an energetic environment, means releasing the denser ideas of a biological singular world and self-view. Physical matter, the perspective of dense and solid objects is an illusion of the senses. Your physical senses are calibrated, your entire physical system is designed to participate in the illusion of physicality, for the full joy of the physical experience.

Your sensory system filters out more information second by second than is conceivable to your conscious mind. You do not perceive all that there is to perceive through your limited senses. You but access a very small spectrum or field of information out of all that is available and active in the Unified Whole. There are certain creatures in your world that see more than you do, that hear more than you do, that feel more than you do, that sense more than you do.

There are human beings in your world that look out through their physical senses and access and download much more information than is thought to be ordinary or normal. They do so because there is more to your world and environment than you currently allow yourself to experience. There is much more to your own being than you currently allow yourself to access and live. And although your senses from your current perspective give the illusion of solidity, not a single aspect of you is as solid as you perceive or believe, and not a single part of you is a gathering of hard unchanging physical solid matter.

There is nothing about your reality that is in a word "physical".

Well-being in its Infinite form is absolute to your reality, and by tuning into and mobilizing ideas vibrating at a higher frequency, you will step into a higher frequency domain simultaneously active to the one you are currently experiencing, and experience physical well-being as your dominant state. You will change your own vibration. You will change the spin and velocity of the consciousness that you are. You will give yourself access to a new reality, to a new world, to a Universe you have not allowed yourself to shift into until now. Your own physical system is the greatest quantum mechanical creative device you will ever encounter. All of your experiences are as possible as your beliefs allow them to be. All of your experiences are reflectors of the ideas you have programmed yourself with, that you have encoded your cellular and vibrational template of being with.

Every idea you hold of what disease is and illness is, is based on the outdated paradigm of there existing factors outside of you. Up until now you may have believed that diseases, viruses, and the various illnesses that take shape in the physical body are something apart from you, from who and what you are.

What you will now realize as you take yourself through the stream of consciousness made available to you through this book is that everything is an expression of who you are in this moment, who you take yourself to be in this moment. You only experience who and what you are conscious of being. You only experience the world that you believe exists. You only actualize and manifest into your body-Universe reality what you believe is true, possible, and valid.

Even that which you perceive to be illness and disease is your own creative self-expression. That you observe into being the diseases that manifest in your physical system, your body-mind apparatus, will be crystal clear to you, for there is nothing else and no one else creating in your personal reality. There is nothing else and no one else observing experiences into your body-Universe reality. There is nothing else and no one else believing your beliefs for you, running your faulty programs for you. *You are the sole author of all that you make manifest in and as your physical experience.*

What you create as your physical experience, what you create as your physical body is entirely up to you and the vibratory ideas you tune into to make manifest. Whatever you believe to be true and valid will make itself known in your experience. Beliefs are self-perpetuating entities. Installed ideas like to validate themselves by expressing in and through you. You do not experience a reality, you experience the reality you believe is possible. You do not experience your world as it is, you only experience your world as you are – as you have programmed yourself to be. And if you believe in a reality where the body operates and behaves in a certain way (i.e. with the "normal" occurrence of disease), then it is that expected outcome which you will experience.

You are the sole author of all that you make manifest in and as your body-Universe reality.

VII.   REDEFINING DIS-EASE

All illness from your "common" cold and aches or pains, to what you consider to be deadly manifestations in your physical body, are ideas, unique wave-forms, you have agreed upon and have integrated into your reality-creating platform. You have assumed that the definitions you have been given on these appearances are the only definitions that exist. You have assumed that there is only one definition to the patterns of energy that form in your reality. And it is these agreed upon definitions that make themselves known to you in your day to day experience as the various undesirable circumstances and conditions that manifest through or in your physical body.

There is nothing in your physical time-space reality that has only one definition. Nothing is as it appears to be. No appearance or manifestation is as it appears to be. Nothing is ever just what you think it is. All information that appears is neutral in nature. Energy is vast and unformed until you collapse it into being in your world through yourself. You are the sole definer of all that manifests in your world, in your view. You are the molder of the clay of life. And you have the power to change your definitions anytime you choose so that you can experience something different, a new possibility, a new form. You are the Light Maker, the Alchemist, of your world.

What physical beings translate as experiences of diseases or illnesses are only indicators of resistance to the natural flow of the energy that creates this physical Universe. Your entire physical Universe is light and information, patterns of energy vibrating at a specific frequency and crystallizing to form as the physical body and Universe that you perceive. When there is resistance to this flow, there is a distortion in the way the information that is constantly flowing through your physical apparatus is encoded in and as your physical body. It is this distortion that is translated and experienced as dis-ease. It is the feedback that universal power is not flowing freely because of something you are focusing on, that is then physically translated as an experience of symptoms of some dis-ease.

Your physical body and Universe cannot exist without the unreserved flow of Universal Energy. Your body and everything in your view is powered by the endless flow of this Universal Power. This energy that animates your physical reality is constantly and endlessly flowing through all physical systems, and that includes your body. It is any focus on low vibration ideas, thoughts, beliefs that limits this flow, and it is the limited flow of universal power that is then communicated to you as the initial experience of dis-ease. Yet, because you have defined these indicators to be negative, you have created them to be much more complex programs that evolve into patterns that continue to limit the flow of Universal Power. Remember, beliefs, ideas, definitions are all self-perpetuating entities. Whatever you believe them to be, however you have defined them to be, they will actualize in that way to validate their existence.

In your physical Universe there is only absolute well-being and a resistance to this absolute well-being. You have trained yourself into resisting the flow of this energizing and animating power by creating and thinking contradictory thoughts, and by taking temporary vibrational indicators to be real, independent occurrences. They are not, and you can now begin to see them in this way. They are only transient indicators of how you're flowing energy, and the only thing that keeps them in place is your insistence and belief that they are in fact real and independent realities unto themselves. The moment you shift such a belief parameter, you give yourself the space to experience these subtle indicators as just that, indicators to re-connect yourself fully to the flow of Universal power.

Make a list of all the diseases you know or have experienced and bring yourself into the recognition that not a single one of these diseases, viruses, or illness, not any one of these manifestations, are real apart from your belief that they are real. You, by your very belief in them, are empowering them into your reality and physical experience. You are the sole author of all that you make manifest in your body-Universe reality. There is not one thing that is not a creation of your own Consciousness-matrix.

All that these diseases are, is evidence of how the beings of your physical system have disallowed the stream of life energy, the stream of absolute well-being. Every disease or illness known to you, every diagnosis that you believe is real and possible, is only vibrational evidence of how someone else, some place else, has disallowed or restricted the flow of life energy through their physical apparatus. And it is the vibrational evidence of another being that you are including and integrating into your own personal experience. Go through your list of diseases and ask yourself when you started believing in the reality of this pattern. For each pattern or disease-program you have installed into your outlook, your perspective, ask yourself when you first became aware of it, when you first became conscious of it and accepted it into yourself.

Every disease known to you or yet to be discovered is an indicator of resistance to well-being, which is an individual choice that need not apply to you and how you flow energy through your physical apparatus. There is only well-being and resistance to this well-being through the limiting thoughts you have practiced into belief patterns, and the realities you have empowered in consensus to the mis-creations or mis-perceptions of other beings. Well-being is the sole reality, all else is the manifestation of your misunderstanding.

All patterns of energy, all consciousness programs, are empowered by you and your belief in them. You are the fuel behind your reality, you are the power behind your experiences. What sustains any occurrence in your physical experience is your belief in the validity and truth of that occurrence. What you believe to be real, will come into your experience, for your belief in its realness is an invitation for that pattern of energy to enter your personal energy field and actualize as a physical experience. What you believe to be real is a program you install into your consciousness-matrix. What you believe, the thoughts you have thought repeatedly and accepted to be true, and what manifests as your body-Universe reality is always a match. And in the absence of vibrational resistance, the patterns of thought that disallow energy to freely flow through your physical apparatus, any and all appearance of disease and discomfort would completely disappear.

You are at all times the sole author of all that you make manifest in and as your body-Universe reality.

40

SECTION II
DAILY EXERCISES

VIII. THE POWER OF PRACTICE

Experiencing yourself and every structure of your multidimensional energetic being as energy and consciousness, is a practice you must engage in daily. It takes repeated exposure and interaction with new ideas to habituate them. It is by repeatedly engaging with these new ideas through consistent practice that you make them available to your conscious awareness. It is your repeated attention to a new idea that solidifies and installs it into your consciousness-matrix. You practiced yourself into the outlook you right now hold. You practiced yourself into seeing yourself as a physical biological being. You thought those thoughts repeatedly until they became knowing's. You practiced yourself into experiencing your being as limited, vulnerable, and susceptible to perceived outside influences.

And so beginning to experience yourself from this new lens of being an energetic being, made up of mostly empty space and vibrating particles, will take practice. Recognizing yourself as a field of consciousness is a lens you must choose to put on consciously until it becomes crystalized as your new outlook. Each day when you re-emerge into your waking world, you reload your attitudes, beliefs, and expectations into your consciousness. These programs, these old and outdated definitions, are active and running even though you may not be consciously aware of them. By consciously integrating and practicing new thought patterns daily based on an energetic model of reality and your identity as consciousness, you can automate these new definitions to serve as your new modes of perception and experience.

    The exercises outlined here will highlight ways for you to begin this practice. Engage with them daily until you find yourself naturally doing them without conscious thought – until they become your default modes of operation. Just like driving a car, or tying your shoe lace, everything you engage in within your world is something you first had to practice before developing it into an easy habit you never had to consciously think to do again. It is the same here. Until you stabilize in accessing this new Universe, this new energetic platform, consciously engage with these practices and any other that you come across that resonate with you so that they become second nature to you. They will become second nature to you.

IX. BODY SCAN

Take a moment at the beginning of each day, before getting out of bed, to slowly run your awareness through your entire physical body. This only takes about three to five minutes to do but the benefits are measureless.

Begin with the top of your head and slowly move your awareness down to your toes resting your awareness at various points in the body. You can use the name of a specific body part to anchor your attention in that area, or you can use your right hand to guide you to different points on the body, before moving down to the next region. Start with the top of your head, then gently move your awareness and attention down to your eyes, then your nose, lips, neck, shoulders, chest, waist, hands, belly, hips, pelvis, thighs, rear, knees, calves, ankles, and toes breathing slowly and naturally. Then move back up to the top of your head anchoring at each key area.

If you find your attention wandering away with thoughts, simply bring your awareness back to the last point you remember and continue with your body scan.

This exercise is a gentle energy massage you give to your physical system. Every cell, every muscle tissue, every layer of your physical system benefits from your open attention to it. Energy flow follows your attention, so whatever part of your body you focus on in this way is receiving the cleansing benefits of pure energy, pure universal power. Your cells, tissues, and deep into your bones are all revitalized, cleansed, and energized. This is a great way to release resistance, tension, and stagnation and restore the balanced flow of energy in and through your physical system. And it is something you can do anytime, anywhere. It is also a great way to center yourself, to withdraw thought out of the mind and into the body for a moment of mental rest and quietness.

Releasing Resistance is a moment to moment choice that you can make at the start of your day with this daily exercise. You can choose to step into your day with ease and openness.

X. ENERGY WORK

For the most part, your practiced habit is to reach for physical solutions anytime you experience any kind of a discomfort. Your practiced habit has been to research or search for names of illnesses, definitions of diseases, symptoms of problems. While such practices serve you for a biological physical world view, from an energetic standpoint they do not offer you energetic solutions. If you are to begin using an energetic model of reality and experience yourself as consciousness, then you must begin to engage with practices that treat everything in your world as patterns of light and information – not symptoms and definitions, but simple vibrational data and simple energetic feedback.

You exist in a sea of energy, and this energy is flooding the physical body from every direction moment after moment. And all that manifests as an imbalance of any kind is indicating that this flow of energy has been obstructed. There are many energy balancing tools available to you that you can incorporate into your daily experience. Tools like Reiki, Tai Chi, Qi Gong, Matrix Energetics, Yuen Method, Quantum Entrainment and more all allow you to engage with yourself as an energetic structure, or at least have a focus on the power and benefit of energy flow for your physical apparatus, your body. These can be very useful to you in your shift in consciousness. The more you integrate any tool or practice that emphasizes the energetic nature and power of your own being, that puts forth an energetic model of reality, into your everyday experience, the more you accelerate your shift in consciousness into perceiving and experiencing yourself and your world as energy.

    If you haven't already, look into any one of them and see what you can take away and incorporate into your own daily practice. You can do all and any kind of energy alignment for yourself, on your own physical body. Every energy meridian, every point of energy flow, exists within you as it does in all other beings. There is nothing less energetic about you. There is nothing less vibrational about you. The only difference maybe the level of practice interacting with yourself as an energy being and so the level of openness to receiving and flowing universal power freely. If you are so pulled to do so, you can also find practitioners either locally in your region or through remote/distance assistance to assist you into coming into alignment with universal power. Make working with your body as an energetic system ordinary for yourself.

XI. CONTEMPLATE DAILY THOUGHT

In Section III of this book, you are offered a daily stream of thought. Allow yourself to contemplate and consider these ideas. Marinate in them. Write them out or translate them into your own understanding. Let yourself integrate your own version of these ideas into your consciousness. Like all other things, the beliefs you hold are practiced patterns of thought. So let yourself practice what you understand from the stream of consciousness made available to you through this book

Every idea you entertain vibrates at a specific frequency, every idea you are offered vibrates at a unique frequency, and as you focus on that idea, you activate it within yourself. It becomes a frequency you generate within the Consciousness that you are. It is this activated pattern of energy that is the basis of your physical reality. The higher the ideas you entertain, the more flexible and malleable your physical reality, which includes your body, becomes. The universe you engage in and the ideas you hold are always a match, so these daily thoughts offered here serve as a bridge into your new world, your new way of experiencing your body and your sense of well-being.

You author your physical experience through the thoughts you anchor and encode into your Consciousness-matrix. The frequencies you generate in response to these thoughts will travel a great length to have you experience the shift in consciousness, the shift in reality, the shift into a new Universe and way of experiencing well-being.

You are the sole author of all that you make manifest in and as your body-Universe reality.

XII.   PRACTICE PRESENCE

What you experience as presence, that sense of simply being aware and present, is the only thing in this reality that is not a program you are running, which is not a program of consciousness. That bears repeating. The only reality in your waking world that is not a program, installed information, is the awareness of simply Being Here Now. Your primal state, the foundation of all that you experience in this reality emerges first out of your sense of being here now. This awareness of being you access in this immediate moment is beyond space and beyond time, it is beyond all the aspects of your waking world.

All there is, is this One eternal moment, there is no other moment. This immediate space of Now-ness contains within it all the infinite possible moments that have ever been or will ever come to be. Just as in your movie theater there is but one screen upon which countless frames are displayed in continuity, it is on the backdrop of this One eternal moment that the sequence of frames that you experience as your waking world are displayed.

The state that you experience as presence, as fully being anchored in the eternal Now is an expanded state of consciousness. When consciousness contracts mind and the world arise. When consciousness expands, all things dissolve and the eternal Now makes itself known. In vibrational terms you can understand expansion as an increase in the speed of vibration of consciousness or entering a higher octave of being, while contraction is a decrease in speed of vibration of consciousness or emerging to a lower octave or tone of being.

Linear time, the sense of having a past and future, is only a thought streams you are tuning into and empowering in your powerful Now-moment. They are programs, belief patterns you pick up and install into your consciousness matrix. Past and future are only thoughts that you are thinking. The past and the future are only a story you are telling right here and right now. Many of your great teachers have long taught you that the past and the future are pure mental fabrications. Take a moment to test this out for yourself. Right where you are in this moment, how are you accessing anything that came "before" right now? How are you accessing anything that comes "after" this immediate moment?

Take a moment to notice what you are experiencing as you answer those questions. Notice how it's all thought and mental pictures? The only time is here. The only place is Now. You cannot negate in any way the experience of this immediate moment, the space of Now that contains all that appears in and as your world in this instant. Anything prior to or beyond this moment is completely imaginary – it is simply an experience of the image-making power of the mind. Test it out. Beyond this immediate moment, all that you encounter is the movement of your own mind, and nothing else. Mental movement is useful for accomplishing goals and desires in your reality, but the trap of linear perception, of weaving a past and a future to your immediate reality is that you perpetuate limiting programs into your every Now-moment.

So the practice of presence, the practice of bringing yourself into the simple awareness of just being present in your Now-moment is integral to you fully accessing the infinite well of well-being that is here right now. In your residing in this moment as pure presence, you allow yourself to not only receive more energy flow, more information, not only do you open yourself up to insights and inspired ideas, but you also allow yourself to observe more. You allow yourself to expand to receive and observe more than you would were you contracted into the realm of the mind.

At the start of each day anchor your full attention in the fullness of your immediate moment. *Nothing came before Here. Nothing happened before Now.* Let that be your anchoring mantra. Keep noticing how what you experience as past and future are simply images your mind is generating. Keep returning your attention to simply being aware without moving with the contents that arise in your being aware.

This will allow you to expand into the ever-present Stillness within you. It will help you to release whatever resistant thought-stream of your now imagined yesterdays and tomorrows that you have activated within you. It will help you to release all that came before this moment. It will help you to release all that you think will come after this moment. And it will allow you to embody and merge into the cleansing frequency of *That* which you translate as Stillness, as Presence.

It's a powerful practice.

XIII. POSITIVE FOCUS

Conditioned thinking, your habituated mode of thinking, often focuses on what's going wrong with your physical system. You seldom ask yourself or are asked by those in your experience "what's right with you?" Make it your practice to each day make note of what's going right with your physical system. How has your body been serving you? What's working perfectly in your physical body? What's right with your physical being?

Negative focus, the habituated focus on what's going wrong or could go wrong with your physical system, is resistant. Such a focus naturally interferes with the flow of life energy through the physical system. Such a focus cuts off the energy the physical body needs to remain in balance. Such a focus creates interference patterns. Such a focus closes your reception channels and creates blockages. Such a focus is what ultimately manifests as discomfort and dis-ease in your physical apparatus. There is only well-being or resistance to it.

Allowing yourself to focus on the positive aspects not only immediately shifts the energy you generate within yourself and attune to, but it also opens up all of your channels of reception and releases the contraction and tension points that were being formed in the body because of resistance. It naturally restores the flow of energy through your countless meridians. A positive focus is cleansing, energizing, and rejuvenating to all parts of your physical system. You are your own temple of rejuvenation.

With a little consistent practice of deliberate

positive focus, you will naturally lift off of the resistant patterns of thought that you have normalized and experience the benefits of keeping yourself in an open and receptive state to the life energy that is constantly and abundantly flowing to you.

So practice and habituate your ability to focus on what's right with the physical system. Feel how it feels to focus on what's flowing and functioning perfectly. Feel how all the muscles and cells of the body respond to such a focus. Make lists. Think about it. Dwell on it. Marinate in it. Practice it.

XIV. APPRECIATE! APPRECIATE! APPRECIATE!

The energy you experience when you are in a state of appreciation is one of the fastest moving energy streams available to you. Make it a habit to step into the stream of appreciation frequently, if not daily.

Create a *Book of Appreciation* for yourself that you can write into at the start and end of your day. Keep it on your nightstand or underneath your pillow. Keep it within reach and make it your dominant intent to exercise and flex your appreciation muscle. Whatever you appreciate, you exponentially empower. Whatever you appreciate, you magnetize to continue to appear in your experience. Everything you appreciate has a tendency to return to you tenfold. Use your power of appreciation as you would ritually use the brush for your hair or teeth. The time you spend appreciating will do more for your body-Universe reality than any physical action you participate in.

What do you appreciate about your physical system?
What do you appreciate about your health?
What do you appreciate about various aspects of your physical life?

Tuning into such a high frequency at the start and end of your day absolutely ensures that you are starting your emergence into waking consciousness in an open and receptive mode.

XV.   DAILY RELEASE

Releasing resistance is key to keeping your physical system at its optimal functioning. The more at ease you are about your moments, the more you keep yourself in a relaxed and flexible state of mind, the less blockages, stagnation, and tension you create in your physical system – the less contraction you bring about of your energy meridians.

Resistance is not created all at once. It is the culmination of the little frustrations you allow to arise in your awareness and hold on to from moment to moment. Resistance is a gradual buildup of thoughts vibrating at a low frequency. It is a clogging up of your energy channels by accumulated low frequency dense patterns of energy ("bad" feeling thoughts).

When you let your contractions of consciousness, contractions of meridians, go unchecked and unreleased, you accumulate packets of dense patterns in your energy field, in your personal energy-matrix. So it is these packets you want to dissolve, cleanse, and let go of. The more attentive you are to the reality within yourself, in your mind and in your body, the more easily you will be able to keep yourself open and tuned in to the flow of universal power.

Make it your intention and practice to completely release all that came before the moment you stepped into your bed to sleep. Let yourself withdraw from waking consciousness on the note of total ease, release, and freedom. Make it your deliberate practice to release the mental story you've built up during the course of your day. Your mind picks up where it leaves off. If you are slightly agitated before sleep, that's the state of mind and pattern of energy waiting for you when you emerge back into waking consciousness. Allow yourself to tune into and see what needs releasing before you fall asleep. Release those little frustrations, judgments, and quiet criticisms that have built up in your day.

SECTION III
THE WORKBOOK

INSTRUCTIONS

Each day contains a stream of thought for you to contemplate followed by exercises for you to take part in as you go on about your day. There is a daily process you take yourself through over the course of 40 days. If the ideas offered in this book are new for you, you can take yourself through the these streams of thoughts multiple times and repeat the process until you feel the shift in consciousness within yourself. You will feel the change.

Ideally you'll do these process first thing in the morning so that you begin to tune into and steer yourself toward this higher-frequency field of perception when your mind or brain waves are still in receptive mode. For the same reason, it's ideal to continue these processes right before you go to sleep. Processing information when your brain/mind is least active and preoccupied, means you'll be able to give this material the kind of relaxed attention that's necessary to make a shift in your consciousness.

You may wonder why 40 days. It takes repeated exposure to an idea to solidify and integrate that new idea into your consciousness-matrix. It is through repeated contact with new ideas that they become familiar and second-nature to you. When you consistently give a new idea your attention, you flow energy into that idea until it is dense enough for it to be integrated into your conscious outlook. Repetition is and has been the pattern of everything you've learned. Everything you right now know with full certainty is an idea you've repeatedly entertained and accepted. What was once just an idea, now is solid knowledge to you. So the integration process requires your unbroken attention for a given period of time. Both in the traditions of the East and the West, 40 days is held to be the length of time necessary to set such a transformation into motion. And so that rule-set is being applied to these exercises also. It's important that you go through these streams of thought with perfect continuity at least the first time through so that you can build up an energetic momentum and attune to the stream of consciousness offered in this book.

Engage yourself in these thought streams daily. Commit to change your inner template. Do all the exercises and allow yourself to dwell on and practice the new thoughts you are offered. Tune in to this stream of consciousness frequently. For as you do, you will encode your consciousness-matrix with higher-frequency patterns of information and so begin to think and experience your physical well-being in a completely new way.

Things you'll need:
1. This book.
2. Your firm decision to shift.
3. A writing journal to process this information, practice turning into the new streams of consciousness, and keep a record of your insights.

SUGGESTED GUIDELINES

1) As a rule, it's important to keep your deliberate effort to shift your consciousness on your chosen subject to yourself. Keep it as your secret so as not to introduce the negative patterns of thought active in other's into your efforts. This is your work and yours alone so mind the kind of input you allow into your efforts. Be mindful of who and in what way you share your decision to make the internal shift with.

2) These efforts aren't about making anything happen. You no more have to make what you're wanting happen than you have to pull the grass out of the ground or manually rotate the earth on its axis. There are natural laws at work here and you are merely working with those laws by releasing your practiced patterns of resistance. You really don't need to hammer anything into place so let your focus be soft, let your focus only be on changing your patterns of thought, shifting your vibration, redefining your inner template. And you do this not for some outcome, but just to shift. The natural outcome of fulfillment is an inevitability.

3) Keep conscious note that appreciation of all the things you already have on every subject is the quickest way to open your energy channels and increase the flow of the creative powerful energy of the Universe into your experience. Resistance in the way of critical thoughts, doubtful thoughts,

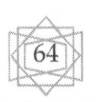

and the like only serve to block or pinch off the flow of Universal energy. Let your day to day mantra be: Appreciate! Appreciate! Appreciate!

4) Keep your attention on the Cause of everything you experience. Do not be swayed by the outcomes, the conditions currently manifested in and around your body-Universe reality. All conditions and circumstances are rapidly changing right in this instant, they are dissolving in the instant you decide to flow your energy elsewhere. Remember, everything around you and swirling within you is light and information – it is all vibration, it is all energy. The Cause of it all is always your own Consciousness, and the thoughts you have encoded yourself with. Resolve to work at the level of this Cause. Remind yourself that you are the sole author of all that you make manifest in and as your body-Universe reality.

5) Relieve yourself from determining or deciding how your shift in consciousness will manifest. The HOW is none of your business. Allow the infinite intelligence of the Universe, the very same intelligence that has brought you to this brilliant point of being in this world, from its broader all-seeing vantage point, to flow it to you through easy and accessible channels. It's not your work to figure out "how" anything will come to you or materialize into your view. Your only job is to manage the thoughts you radiate, how you vibrate, and then get out of the way.

6) Remind yourself that fulfillment and absolute well-being in all aspects of your life, is your birthright for the simple reason that you exist. You are designed to thrive. There is absolutely nothing that you cannot become or materialize. "Impossible" is not a word or concept known by the Intelligence that builds this Universe. Line yourself up to that omni-possibility. If life, if this Universe has inspired you to conceive of a desire, that desire can absolutely materialize. There are no exceptions.

7) Take *time* out of the equation. The only place is Here and the only time is Now. Welcome yourself to the eternal space of Creation. Whatever your desire, it can only materialize in the Now. There is no future moment. There is no future time of tomorrow, later, or "in six months" for your desire to be visible to you. The only place and time for it to materialize, is right here and right now. Be mindful of the mental tendency to futurize and set up a condition of future-time for materialization. Now is all there is. Time is a factor only you can introduce into your body-Universe reality.

8) Think of this 40 day process as a way to "upgrade" your mental operating system. It's really not anything more mystical or abstract. You're simply re-writing the thoughts you've embedded or programmed your mind with up until now. You are the magic and miracle of the Universe. There is nothing outside of you

creating in your reality.

9) Be consistent and be patient with yourself and your practice. It takes a buildup of energy in Consciousness to materialize into the physical so let your intention be to make that necessary shift in Consciousness. Allow yourself to take in information along the lines of creating change from the inside out. There are endless resources and information available that you can make use of to fill your mind with the type of thoughts necessary to make such a shift. Immerse yourself in this understanding so that you can consistently tune out of the old limiting beliefs you have trained yourself to hold as real and valid.

10) Bring yourself to keep focusing on what it is that you do want. Decide to supply and apply your power, your energy only to what it is you're wanting to see moment to moment. Commit to yourself and your vision. Say to yourself each day "today, no matter where I go or what I do, I choose to flow my energy only to those things I am wanting. I choose my vision." You are always radiating the energy of the thing that has your attention the most, so let what captivates you be the thing that you want.

You are the sole author of all that you make manifest in and as your body-Universe reality.

STREAM 1: THE TIMELESS PERFECTION OF YOUR PHYSICAL BODY

The energy that manifests as your physical body and universe is in a state of timeless perfection. The substance of the universe does not fluctuate in its abundant and continuous flow. Well-being is absolute and endless at all times, and it is this stream of absolute well-being that creates your entire physical Universe. Your physical body is no exception.

It isn't the energy itself that creates and manifests as disturbances in your physical body but rather your resistance to this pure energy. Your resistance to it in the form of old beliefs and your alignment with these erroneous beliefs is all that materializes as the various physical discomforts that you experience in your personal reality.

You believe that sickness is a natural part of physical experience. You believe that you are vulnerable to "outside" factors. You believe that your health and well-being is in the hands of factors outside of you. You believe that viruses and bacteria and infections are something other than information you tune into and integrate into yourself. You believe that diseases and illness are real and unavoidable aspects of physical experience. You have set up for yourself belief-templates that are in alignment with the absence of well-being.

And so you create for yourself a physical experience that is loyal to the belief-templates you have set up.

QUESTIONS TO ANSWER IN YOUR JOURNAL:

What do you currently believe about yourself and your world?

What is your current identity – who and what are you aware of being?

What is the physical body to you?

How do you define your experiences of dis-ease? What did you used to believe about the cause for dis-ease in the body?

Are you willing to challenge your negative assumptions and belief that an absence of absolute well-being is possible?

Daily Process

- Body Scan – first thing in the morning scan your physical body.
- Contemplate today's consciousness stream – allow yourself to visit today's thought and contemplate the idea presented to you. Come back to this idea frequently throughout your day. Write out your own translation of this stream, your initial impressions and feelings about it.
- Be Present with your Being – allow yourself to be anchored in your powerful Now-consciousness.
- Positive Aspects – let yourself dwell on all that is going RIGHT with your physical system today.
- Appreciate! Appreciate! Appreciate! - allow yourself to tune into the cleansing, rejuvenating, and revitalizing power of the energy you

physically experience in your state of appreciation.
- Release Resistance – before you withdraw from waking consciousness into your dream and sleep state, make it your intention to release whatever minor resistance you may have accumulated or created within your physical system on this day.

STREAM 2: YOU ARE PURE VIBRATION

Your entire physical apparatus, the body you perceive and experience as a mass of hard matter, is entirely vibrational. It is energy. It is light and information. It is predominately empty space. It is barely there. In the words of mystical thought, it is an illusion, a hallucination of your physical brain-body system itself.

Even as you read these words, what you interpret as your physical environment and body, is a reading of frequencies, a registration of electrical stimuli that your holographic brain translates as physical objects located in time and space. Your physical body and brain acts as a quantum device that generates the seemingly physical body-Universe you experience.

The way your physical body feels in any given moment is an indication of the frequencies, the wave-patterns in the form of thoughts and beliefs, you have calibrated it to tune into. Your physical body is reflecting to you the balance of the frequencies you have recorded or encoded upon it. And the higher the frequency of the thought-streams you tune into, the more flexible your experience of your physical body and Universe becomes.

There is nothing about your physical body that is hard solid matter. You are particles waving, and waves appearing and disappearing in a reality composed of energy in motion. Let yourself dwell in this stream for a moment, let yourself dwell on the notion: I *am particles waving, and waving appearing and disappearing in a reality composed of energy in motion.*

QUESTIONS TO ANSWER IN YOUR JOURNAL:

Are you ready to see your whole being as energy? What does an energetic identity mean to you? How does it feel to you to see yourself as being compose of moving particles and empty space?

Are you open to allowing yourself to release the erroneous belief system that you are something other than a being of pure energy, of pure light and vibrational information?

Daily Process
- Body Scan – first thing in the morning scan your physical body.
- Contemplate today's consciousness stream – allow yourself to visit today's thought and contemplate the idea presented to you. Come back to this idea frequently throughout your day. Write out your own translation of this stream, your initial impressions and feelings about it.
- Be Present with your Being – allow yourself to be anchored in your powerful Now-consciousness.
- Positive Aspects – let yourself dwell on all that is going RIGHT with your physical system today.
- Appreciate! Appreciate! Appreciate! - allow yourself to tune into the cleansing, rejuvenating, and revitalizing power of the energy you physically experience in your state of appreciation.
- Release Resistance – before you withdraw from

waking consciousness into your dream and sleep state, make it your intention to release whatever minor resistance you may have accumulated or created within your physical system on this day.

STREAM 3: YOU HAVE QUANTUM ACCESS

In this powerful-Now, this immediate instant, you have quantum access to a powerful reservoir of pure energy, the very energy that constructs your physical body and universe. Past and future, what you perceive as having come before this instant and coming after this instant are mental fabrications. You have access in this instant to tune into a new possibility for your physical body and system, a possibility that your recollection and attachment to what you perceive as the "past" does not allow you to see.

You need not continue creating and mentally validating an undesirable physical condition in this instant. The moment you recognize that the condition you were tuning into is only one possible information stream you were empowering, you give yourself permission to tune out of this information, to cease believing in its reality. As you do, you make a quantum shift, a shift from the very root of all that you experience, to materialize a physical body and Universe in line with what you want to experience.

You, in this Now-moment, are your own temple of rejuvenation and restoration. There is not a single cellular component, there is not a single atom, that is an exception to your ability to shift into a new dimension of physical experience in this very instant. And it is your alignment with the possibility of all that your body can become here and now, that all that your body is in the reality of absolute and unfailing well-being, that will allow you to tap into the quantum field of your physical body and universe to materialize a physical body-Universe you prefer.

All the power you will ever have to alter your experience of physicality, you have right in this immediate instant. There is no other time or point in space in which for you to make the decisive shift.

What do you decide?

QUESTIONS TO ANSWER IN YOUR JOURNAL:

Are you willing to shift into the reality of absolute well-being in this instant?

Are you open to the recognition that you are choosing what information-stream you are tuning into and making valid to your physical experience?

Are you open to choosing anew in this instant?

Are you willing to let go of whatever you think and believe came before this moment?

Daily Process

- Body Scan – first thing in the morning scan your physical body.
- Contemplate today's consciousness stream – allow yourself to visit today's thought and contemplate the idea presented to you. Come back to this idea frequently throughout your day. Write out your own translation of this stream, your initial impressions and feelings about it.
- Be Present with your Being – allow yourself to be anchored in your powerful Now-consciousness.
- Positive Aspects – let yourself dwell on all that is going RIGHT with your physical system today.

- Appreciate! Appreciate! Appreciate! - allow yourself to tune into the cleansing, rejuvenating, and revitalizing power of the energy you physically experience in your state of appreciation.
- Release Resistance – before you withdraw from waking consciousness into your dream and sleep state, make it your intention to release whatever minor resistance you may have accumulated or created within your physical system on this day.

STREAM 4: ALLOWING RECEPTION

Every single atom that makes up your physical body is conscious and aware of its needs. Every atom that vibrates as your physical system is a living conscious intelligence. It is the atoms of your physical body that summon the energy they need to maintain balance and equilibrium. You have never had to think about or plan for how much oxygen is needed to keep the body active. You have never had to think about how much power is needed to keep your hair or nails growing. Every part of your body already knows what it needs and draws to itself the necessary elements. Your body is a self-regulating conscious mechanism composed of intelligent atoms whose natural intention is to remain aligned with absolute well-being, the True Nature of the Intelligence that constructs and supports all aspects of your body-Universe reality.

You, as the identity making use of the physical body have created a web of belief patterns that interfere with the transmission and reception of universal power, energy, between these atoms and the Source Field. And it is these belief patterns that cause resistance which then manifests as symptoms of dis-ease. Your intelligent body is designed to maintain its own balance and to indicate to you whether the balance of your practiced thoughts is in line with well-being or resistant to it. To allow reception begin to deliberately align yourself with, and tune into, thought-streams and events that generate positive feelings within you. Remember, positive feelings are indicating to you that energy is flowing through your physical apparatus in an unrestricted manner – that you are completely plugged in to the flow of universal power.

In short, when you are in full connection to well-being and allowing energy to flow freely through your physical system, you feel good. What you translate as good feelings are your constant indicators that energy is flowing freely and without obstruction through your physical system. When you are resisting well-being and pinching off the flow of Universal Power, you feel low or "bad" - this feeling of lowness is indicating to you that the pure energy of the Universe that supports your physical reality is not freely flowing through your physical brain-body system. Your feelings are constantly indicating to you whether or not you are open and allowing energy to flow freely through your physical being.

Allow to be guided by the emotions that arise within you in each moment. Your physical body is designed with the perfect real-time indicators of how pure energy is flowing through the body in any given moment. Just like your vehicles, your body has the built-in capability of monitoring and indicating the flow of fuel within it - the flow of pure energy!

QUESTIONS TO ANSWER IN YOUR JOURNAL:

Do you recognize and acknowledge the intelligence of your physical system, the intelligence of every cell, every atom that constructs your brain-body apparatus?

What does it mean to you to have an intelligent physical mechanism?

Daily Process

- Body Scan – first thing in the morning scan your physical body.

- Contemplate today's consciousness stream – allow yourself to visit today's thought and contemplate the idea presented to you. Come back to this idea frequently throughout your day. Write out your own translation of this stream, your initial impressions and feelings about it.
- Be Present with your Being – allow yourself to be anchored in your powerful Now-consciousness.
- Positive Aspects – let yourself dwell on all that is going RIGHT with your physical system today.
- Appreciate! Appreciate! Appreciate! - allow yourself to tune into the cleansing, rejuvenating, and revitalizing power of the energy you physically experience in your state of appreciation.
- Release Resistance – before you withdraw from waking consciousness into your dream and sleep state, make it your intention to release whatever minor resistance you may have accumulated or created within your physical system on this day.

STREAM 5: INSTALLING BELIEFS

Every belief you integrate into your consciousness matrix, every belief you accept without question, is like a program you install to automatically run in your physical reality. Whatever belief you accept to be real, true, and valid, will reinforce itself by manifesting in and as your physical experience. It will validate itself. Beliefs are self-perpetuating and self-reinforcing programs that are receiving their power to manifest in your physical experience directly from you. It is your acceptance of them as true and valid that empowers them into manifestation. You, the consciousness that you are, are the only power in your experience.

You can choose to un-install the flawed beliefs of sickness and diseases by recognizing that everything that materializes in and as your physical universe is a result of the beliefs you have empowered into actualization. Nothing is real unless you say it is real. Nothing is true unless you say it's true. There is no pattern of energy or information that asserts itself into your experience without your permission and agreement to participate in that pattern of information. Consciousness is the only power, consciousness is the only reality, consciousness is the only thing operating in and as your reality.

QUESTIONS TO ANSWER IN YOUR JOURNAL:

Are you willing to recognize how unnatural the very idea of sickness and disease are to a reality based on the premise of absolute and unfailing well-being?

Are you ready to release the beliefs that perpetuate the

misconception that it is "normal" to become ill or sick?
Can you acknowledge for yourself that consciousness is the sole cause of all that you experience?

Daily Process

- Body Scan – first thing in the morning scan your physical body.
- Contemplate today's consciousness stream – allow yourself to visit today's thought and contemplate the idea presented to you. Come back to this idea frequently throughout your day. Write out your own translation of this stream, your initial impressions and feelings about it.
- Be Present with your Being – allow yourself to be anchored in your powerful Now-consciousness.
- Positive Aspects – let yourself dwell on all that is going RIGHT with your physical system today.
- Appreciate! Appreciate! Appreciate! - allow yourself to tune into the cleansing, rejuvenating, and revitalizing power of the energy you physically experience in your state of appreciation.
- Release Resistance – before you withdraw from waking consciousness into your dream and sleep state, make it your intention to release whatever minor resistance you may have accumulated or created within your physical system on this day.

STREAM 6: IMMEDIATE SHIFTS

The Unified Source Field in which you exist and experience your physical reality contains all possible outcomes for every aspect of your physical experience. Every possible version of your physical body exists in this instant in its own frequency domain. Every possible state of being exists in your immediate instant. Creation is complete – the infinite sea of possibilities is all here in this moment.

The only place is Here and the only time is Now. Linear time is an illusion. Transformation, restoration, and rejuvenation are not time-bound states of being that you gradually experience but immediate frequency domains you can tune into in your powerful-eternal-Now. You can shift into the frequency domain in which all evidence of disease and discomfort is non-existent if you give yourself the unconditional permission to tune into that frequency domain in your powerful Now, this immediate instant in which you are aware and present.

When you can unequivocally tune into the thought *"the version of me that I am right now is in a completely balanced and resistance free state of being"* you have altered the reality matrix you are participating in – you have shifted yourself into the body-Universe reality of total health and well-being. The amount of time it takes for you to shift from sickness to wellness is the amount of time it takes you to unequivocally tune into the desired outcome that already exists in your powerful Now moment. Immerse yourself in the reality of well-being, let it be the only thing that you see active and alive all around you.

Time is only a condition you place upon

yourself. Time is only a rule-set you have imposed upon your ability to experience your Core Nature of absolute and timeless well-being. Time is not outside of consciousness, time exists only within the consciousness that you are. So you have the ability to take time completely out of the equation.

QUESTIONS TO ANSWER IN YOUR JOURNAL:
Are you willing to release the belief that it takes "time" to experience your well-being?

Are you willing to release the perception that wellness is a state that gradually appears rather than an immediate possibility you can access in your powerful Now?

Daily Process
- Body Scan – first thing in the morning scan your physical body.
- Contemplate today's consciousness stream – allow yourself to visit today's thought and contemplate the idea presented to you. Come back to this idea frequently throughout your day. Write out your own translation of this stream, your initial impressions and feelings about it.
- Be Present with your Being – allow yourself to be anchored in your powerful Now-consciousness.
- Positive Aspects – let yourself dwell on all that is going RIGHT with your physical system today.
- Appreciate! Appreciate! Appreciate! - allow yourself to tune into the cleansing, rejuvenating, and revitalizing power of the energy you

physically experience in your state of appreciation.
- Release Resistance – before you withdraw from waking consciousness into your dream and sleep state, make it your intention to release whatever minor resistance you may have accumulated or created within your physical system on this day.

STREAM 7: UTILIZING YOUR CREATIVE NOW

The version of you that you are in this instant is only manifesting a continuity of experience because you are continuing to tell the same story, you are continuing to tune into the same frequency domain. Pay attention to the thought-streams you are investing your energy in, that you are believing in and are allowing to continue to run in your awareness. Listen to the content of your own mind, listen to the audio stream actively running on loop within yourself. Yesterday's illness, last year's illness, how you'll feel tomorrow or any other thought-streams of "past" and "future" discomfort is something you are creating Now – it is a stream of thought, a story you are allowing to continue to live within you Now.

The past does not create the present but rather it is this moment, this present instant that is creating the past. Marinate in this shift of perspective for a moment. This moment is not a continuation of some previous moment. There is no such thing as "before". Today is not a continuation of your perceived "yesterday". Yesterday's sickness is something you are creating Now. It is a perception. It is a story, a weaving of thoughts, that you are activating and paying attention to Now. Tomorrow's sickness is something you are creating Now. The continuity of any experience and any condition is something you are generating and empowering Now. The story you are telling in this instant, the thought stream you are empowering in this moment, is what is arranging the frames of your physical reality to look and feel as they look and feel.

Past and future do not exist, all perceived past

experiences are frames you are creating in this instant. Here and Now is the only point of Creation in Consciousness. Here and Now is your absolute eternal point of power to create the reality you prefer. You can in this instant tune into the version of you, the frequency domain in which yesterday's perceived sickness never even came into existence.

QUESTION TO ANSWER IN YOUR JOURNAL:
Can you allow yourself to experience the illusion of continuity?

Can you allow yourself to experience the past and the future as the creations of your powerful eternal Now?

What does it mean to you to see the past and future as a creation of this immediate moment?

Daily Process

- Body Scan – first thing in the morning scan your physical body.
- Contemplate today's consciousness stream – allow yourself to visit today's thought and contemplate the idea presented to you. Come back to this idea frequently throughout your day. Write out your own translation of this stream, your initial impressions and feelings about it.
- Be Present with your Being – allow yourself to be anchored in your powerful Now-consciousness.
- Positive Aspects – let yourself dwell on all that is going RIGHT with your physical system today.
- Appreciate! Appreciate! Appreciate! – allow

yourself to tune into the cleansing, rejuvenating, and revitalizing power of the energy you physically experience in your state of appreciation.

- Release Resistance – before you withdraw from waking consciousness into your dream and sleep state, make it your intention to release whatever minor resistance you may have accumulated or created within your physical system on this day.

STREAM 8: SIMULTANEOUS WELLNESS

The thought-stream and so physical experience of well-being exists simultaneously with the thought-streams of discord and disease. Although only absolute well-being is the sole reality of your Universe, you have created streams of information contradictory to this sole reality. You are free in the reality you create. You are so free that you can contradict and participate in a reality that in no way reflects who you really are.

Everything is a thought-stream you are tuning and calibrating yourself to. What appears right now as your physical reality and body is only a frequency domain you have attuned yourself to, but it is not the only domain of experience available to you Now.

Cease believing that sickness and discomfort are the only reality available to you in this instant. You exist in a Field of Infinite Potential right now containing all possible thought-streams, information-streams, outcomes for you to tune into.

You are a deliberate chooser of the information-streams you will tune into in any given instant.

What will you choose to tune into?

Daily Process
- Body Scan – first thing in the morning scan your physical body.
- Contemplate today's consciousness stream – allow yourself to visit today's thought and contemplate the idea presented to you. Come back to this idea frequently throughout your day. Write out your own translation of this

stream, your initial impressions and feelings about it.
- Be Present with your Being – allow yourself to be anchored in your powerful Now-consciousness.
- Positive Aspects – let yourself dwell on all that is going RIGHT with your physical system today.
- Appreciate! Appreciate! Appreciate! - allow yourself to tune into the cleansing, rejuvenating, and revitalizing power of the energy you physically experience in your state of appreciation.
- Release Resistance – before you withdraw from waking consciousness into your dream and sleep state, make it your intention to release whatever minor resistance you may have accumulated or created within your physical system on this day.

STREAM 9: YOU ARE CREATING IT NOW

The only proof you have of being sick or experiencing discomfort in some past moment is the proof you are creating in this immediate instant. It is a perception you are empowering in your Now. It is a mental image you are tuning into and flowing the power of your attention into right now. All your memories and recollections are simultaneous frames of experience you are tuning into right Now. They are stories you are choosing to tell, thought-streams you are choosing to tune into, mental images you are choosing to flow energy into in this immediate moment.

You have developed a tendency to take mere vibrational indicators, temporary appearances that have become visible to reveal to you whether or not you are allowing universal power to flow freely through you, as proof of the validity of your resistance. What you experience as sickness is only an indicator of resistance, it is not proof that sickness is a stand-alone reality. What you experience as discomfort and dis-ease is only showing up in your body-Universe reality to indicate to you that you are, through whatever you have chosen to focus on in your in-the-moment thoughts and attitudes, closing yourself off to the flow of universal power. But because you have created for yourself the belief that sickness is a reality, you continue to give it a meaningful role in your experience of physicality.

You cannot tune into your valid frames of wellness and manifest your proof of absolute well-being at the same time that you tune into your images of sickness. You are choosing the reality you wish to experience right Now.

QUESTIONS TO ANSWER IN YOUR JOURNAL:

Where are you validating and empowering experiences of resistance?
Where can you right now release points of focus that are slowing down or constricting the free flow of universal power through your physical apparatus?

Daily Process

- Body Scan – first thing in the morning scan your physical body.
- Contemplate today's consciousness stream – allow yourself to visit today's thought and contemplate the idea presented to you. Come back to this idea frequently throughout your day. Write out your own translation of this stream, your initial impressions and feelings about it.
- Be Present with your Being – allow yourself to be anchored in your powerful Now-consciousness.
- Positive Aspects – let yourself dwell on all that is going RIGHT with your physical system today.
- Appreciate! Appreciate! Appreciate! - allow yourself to tune into the cleansing, rejuvenating, and revitalizing power of the energy you physically experience in your state of appreciation.
- Release Resistance – before you withdraw from

waking consciousness into your dream and sleep state, make it your intention to release whatever minor resistance you may have accumulated or created within your physical system on this day.

STREAM 10: YOUR FREEDOM TO BE WELL

Your physical body is only as vulnerable as you believe it is. Your physical body is only as susceptible as you believe it is. As a conscious and self-reflecting organism, you have the power to select and reject information that you know isn't an experience you would like to have. You do not have to include and accept every stream of information that is available into your experience. You no more have to listen to and download every possible program available on your radio or television programs, than you have to listen to and download into your consciousness-matrix every "reality" you are offered in your physical experience. You really do not have to buy every ingredient in the store of your reality!

Everything you are offered in this physical experience is information – everything, every belief and thought-stream is light and information you choose to integrate into your personal reality. Every "evidence" of a reality you are offered is only information for you to sift through and choose to include in your experience of physical reality. Let your mantra be: *I choose what I will experience in my Universe.* Let go of letting your world choose for you and begin to choose for yourself.

You are free to create whatever physical experience you wish to have. You are free to install any template of experience into your consciousness-matrix. You are the decider, the selector, the chooser of what belief-programs, what reality-programs, you will allow to play out in your physical experience. Your freedom to be well is absolute and the choice is always yours. You have the right to say "no, this information does not apply to me." You have the right and the powers to uninstall, delete, and altogether reject any information you choose not to integrate into your body-Universe experience. You are powerful enough to choose what you will install into your reality program!

QUESTIONS TO ANSWER IN YOUR JOURNAL:
Are you willing to be absolutely healthy all the time?
Are you open to the possibility of unfailing health until you remove focus from your current physical apparatus?

Daily Process
- Body Scan – first thing in the morning scan your physical body.
- Contemplate today's consciousness stream – allow yourself to visit today's thought and contemplate the idea presented to you. Come back to this idea frequently throughout your day. Write out your own translation of this stream, your initial impressions and feelings about it.
- Be Present with your Being – allow yourself to be anchored in your powerful Now-consciousness.
- Positive Aspects – let yourself dwell on all that is going RIGHT with your physical system today.
- Appreciate! Appreciate! Appreciate! - allow yourself to tune into the cleansing, rejuvenating, and revitalizing power of the energy you physically experience in your state of appreciation.

- Release Resistance – before you withdraw from waking consciousness into your dream and sleep state, make it your intention to release whatever minor resistance you may have accumulated or created within your physical system on this day.

STREAM 11: YOU CHOOSE NOW

You have the ability to choose which version of your physical body you are going to experience in every moment. Every moment is a fresh beginning. Every immediate instant, every Now in which you find yourself aware of being in this waking world, is a clean slate. *Nothing came before this instant. Nothing happened before Now.* Every story or image your mind offers you about a past lives and continues to actualize itself into your reality only if you allow it to.

Every instant is a new Universe unto itself. Every instant is an opportunity to choose again which physical body and which Universe you are going to open your eyes in. This is the living Grace of Consciousness. Each instant, each frame of experience, offers you unlimited possibilities in what can manifest as your physical body and Universe. You are choosing your reality field, your body-Universe reality, in the ever-present powerful Now. There is no other time and there is no other place to choose again and again what you are willing to experience.

QUESTIONS TO ANSWER IN YOUR JOURNAL:
What reality are you choosing?
What possibility are you embodying?

Daily Process
- Body Scan – first thing in the morning scan your physical body.
- Contemplate today's consciousness stream – allow yourself to visit today's thought and contemplate the idea presented to you. Come

back to this idea frequently throughout your day. Write out your own translation of this stream, your initial impressions and feelings about it.
- Be Present with your Being – allow yourself to be anchored in your powerful Now-consciousness.
- Positive Aspects – let yourself dwell on all that is going RIGHT with your physical system today.
- Appreciate! Appreciate! Appreciate! - allow yourself to tune into the cleansing, rejuvenating, and revitalizing power of the energy you physically experience in your state of appreciation.
- Release Resistance – before you withdraw from waking consciousness into your dream and sleep state, make it your intention to release whatever minor resistance you may have accumulated or created within your physical system on this day.

STREAM 12: YOUR CONSCIOUS POWER

QUESTIONS TO ANSWER IN YOUR JOURNAL:
Who is setting the parameters of your physical experience?
What are you allowing to determine what kind of physical body and experience you have?
Where are you getting your information from?
Who is the decider of your body-Universe reality?
Who is the author of your personal reality?

You have the power to break free from mass consciousness, and the countless agreed upon consensus realities, and determine for yourself how you are going to experience your physical body and world. You do not have to plug into what the masses are plugged into. You do not have to actualize within your personal experience what others have chosen to actualize in theirs. Your ability to discern and discriminate has its purpose, to allow you to choose your world.

Everything in your physical Universe is a materialization of conscious focus. All materialization is the focusing effect of activated beliefs, activate programs, and you have absolute power to choose what beliefs you are going to keep active in your individual consciousness-matrix.

Your conscious power to reject streams of information, wave-patterns offered in your world is your best ally in experiencing your physical body the way you want to experience it.

Daily Process

- Body Scan – first thing in the morning scan your physical body.
- Contemplate today's consciousness stream – allow yourself to visit today's thought and contemplate the idea presented to you. Come back to this idea frequently throughout your day. Write out your own translation of this stream, your initial impressions and feelings about it.
- Be Present with your Being – allow yourself to be anchored in your powerful Now-consciousness.
- Positive Aspects – let yourself dwell on all that is going RIGHT with your physical system today.
- Appreciate! Appreciate! Appreciate! - allow yourself to tune into the cleansing, rejuvenating, and revitalizing power of the energy you physically experience in your state of appreciation.
- Release Resistance – before you withdraw from waking consciousness into your dream and sleep state, make it your intention to release whatever minor resistance you may have accumulated or created within your physical system on this day.

STREAM 13: YOU ARE PURE POWER

Your preferred reality and physical body exists in your immediate space of Now. Whatever event you believe is happening only stays on your screen of experience because you are giving validity to it. You are the power behind your every experience. Your Universe is in existence because you are in existence. You and your physical Universe are not separate occurrences. Your reality is powered by you. Your reality is supported by you. It is your own existence that determines and shapes the reality of your body-Universe experience.

When you take what appears as a vibrational indicator to reveal to you the balance of your thoughts, the dominant frequency you are broadcasting, as a hard fact unchanging reality, you continue to hold that vibrational indicator in place and experience it moment after moment. When you take the materialized event or condition for the transient frequency indicator that it is, your ability to tune into your preferred simultaneous reality will be much more immediate.

You are pure power, and you are doubtlessly the Ultimate Power of your personal reality.

Daily Process
- Body Scan – first thing in the morning scan your physical body.
- Contemplate today's consciousness stream – allow yourself to visit today's thought and contemplate the idea presented to you. Come back to this idea frequently throughout your

day. Write out your own translation of this stream, your initial impressions and feelings about it.
- Be Present with your Being – allow yourself to be anchored in your powerful Now-consciousness.
- Positive Aspects – let yourself dwell on all that is going RIGHT with your physical system today.
- Appreciate! Appreciate! Appreciate! - allow yourself to tune into the cleansing, rejuvenating, and revitalizing power of the energy you physically experience in your state of appreciation.
- Release Resistance – before you withdraw from waking consciousness into your dream and sleep state, make it your intention to release whatever minor resistance you may have accumulated or created within your physical system on this day.

STREAM 14: EVERYTHING IS LIGHT AND INFORMATION

Everything is light and information. The body you perceive to be real is light and information, and what's keeping this pattern of light and information visible to you the way that it appears, is your belief that it is real the way it is. Nothing is as it appears to be in your physical reality. Under the right magnification all that is visible as your Universe is empty space. Stay with that thought for a moment. Everything seemingly visible and solid in your world is primordial Emptiness, the void and source of all creative expression. As your senses are currently calibrated only to perceive a specific spectrum of light, you access but a minuscule amount of data that you experience as your physical Universe. What you perceive as your physical body-Universe is an illusion of your sense-apparatus. Adjust this lens, and you bring yourself to experience a reality that is completely different.

The power of your belief that something is real is the power that supplies energy to the patterns of light that appear as your physical environment. The appearance of your physical body is an illusion, a sensory hallucination, a holographic construction based on the beliefs you have lined up for yourself. You are Pure Consciousness and your belief in your body as real the way it is, creates a reflection of light and information that you decode as physical reality.

Learn to see through the illusion of the wave-patterns and information that appear as your physical body in this instant. Let yourself experience that the body you right now perceive is a pure construction of your brain-body system, your nervous system. Learn to step into the understanding that everything in your physical Universe, including your body, is malleable and subject to instantaneous alterations or change in your preferred direction.

You are the sole author of all that you view in and as your body-Universe reality.

Daily Process
- Body Scan – first thing in the morning scan your physical body.
- Contemplate today's consciousness stream – allow yourself to visit today's thought and contemplate the idea presented to you. Come back to this idea frequently throughout your day. Write out your own translation of this stream, your initial impressions and feelings about it.
- Be Present with your Being – allow yourself to be anchored in your powerful Now-consciousness.
- Positive Aspects – let yourself dwell on all that is going RIGHT with your physical system today.
- Appreciate! Appreciate! Appreciate! - allow yourself to tune into the cleansing, rejuvenating, and revitalizing power of the energy you physically experience in your state of appreciation.
- Release Resistance – before you withdraw from waking consciousness into your dream and sleep state, make it your intention to release whatever minor resistance you may have accumulated or created within your physical system on this day.

STREAM 15: WELL-BEING IS NATURAL

The information you validate by accepting it as true and real is the information that constructs your physical reality. Your reality is a materialization of the information, the wave-patterns, you have activated and empowered through your belief in the realness of them. What you experience are the information patterns you have integrated, installed, into your personal energy field.

If you've incorporated the belief that it is natural for your physical body to experience an uncomfortable breakdown as it gets older, then every single one of your trillions of cells will obey this belief-command. Your body will not contradict you. Your Universe will not behave outside of your reality-margins. What you believe is true, what you believe is possible is what shapes the Universe you experience. Every belief you entertain about the state of your physical body, from the probability of disease and viruses to the probability of physical decline with aging, is a command you give to the conscious intelligent particles that create your physical body. Your body is an interactive intelligence. Your cells are an interactive intelligence. Your entire immediate environment is an interactive intelligence reflecting and obeying the instructions you put in place through your beliefs.

It is natural to experience and materialize your physical well-being throughout your entire experience of physical focus.

QUESTIONS TO ANSWER IN YOUR JOURNAL:
What did you used to believe was a natural physical experience?

Where are you questioning your beliefs now?
What beliefs are you ready to let go of?
What are you willing to experience now as a reality for your physical body?

Daily Process
- Body Scan – first thing in the morning scan your physical body.
- Contemplate today's consciousness stream – allow yourself to visit today's thought and contemplate the idea presented to you. Come back to this idea frequently throughout your day. Write out your own translation of this stream, your initial impressions and feelings about it.
- Be Present with your Being – allow yourself to be anchored in your powerful Now-consciousness.
- Positive Aspects – let yourself dwell on all that is going RIGHT with your physical system today.
- Appreciate! Appreciate! Appreciate! - allow yourself to tune into the cleansing, rejuvenating, and revitalizing power of the energy you physically experience in your state of appreciation.
- Release Resistance – before you withdraw from waking consciousness into your dream and sleep state, make it your intention to release whatever minor resistance you may have accumulated or created within your physical system on this day.

STREAM 16: DELIBERATELY CHOOSING YOUR FREQUENCY RANGE OF EXPERIENCE

Every thought you tune into and encode into your consciousness-matrix belongs to a specific frequency domain, a unique dimension of experience. Just like every radio station or every TV station has its own unique broadcast signal, so do the infinite possible realities, the numberless possible outcomes, available to you. The wave-like nature of your physical Universe and Being means you are not consistently experiencing one frequency domain but rather dipping in and out of multiple frequency fields in direct correlation to the streams of thought you tune into and activate in your consciousness-matrix. You are constantly flipping through your reality channels.

You do not experience physical discomfort in a continuous manner though your selective recollections may deceive you into such a belief. If you paid attention to the flow of your own being in what you experience as a 24-hour cycle, you would see that you do not feel physical discomfort every second of every day, even in what you have called chronic experiences. When you enter the state of deep sleep, when your brain waves reach a certain level, the experience of pain dissolves completely. This should indicate to you the true nature of any kind of discomfort. When the physical system, when your physical nervous system reaches a certain frequency all types of discomfort dissolve.

You are at all times experiencing multiple versions of your universe and physical body. Remember, you exist in a sea of energy that is in constant and continuous flux. Everything about you and around you is flickering in and out of location continuously. The multi-dimensional nature of your Universe and Being further means that you are not experiencing one version of your body and Universe continuously, but rather dipping in and out of, tuning in and out of body-Universe realities of a particular frequency range. As you learn to tune into higher and higher frequency ranges in the Infinite pool of this Vibrational Matrix, your experience of your physical body and personal reality will astound you. Recognizing yourself as an energetic being, recognizing yourself as a field of consciousness, a frequency field of light and information, you are shifting the frequency range of experiences you make available to yourself. And this shift will translate as a shift in the structure and appearance of your seemingly physical world.

Question the seeming continuity of your physical experience.
Question what seems obvious and solid.
Question the way you are experiencing your physical body and world.
Question the very concepts you had held to be true and valid.

Daily Process
- Body Scan – first thing in the morning scan your physical body.
- Contemplate today's consciousness stream – allow yourself to visit today's thought and contemplate the idea presented to you. Come back to this idea frequently throughout your

day. Write out your own translation of this stream, your initial impressions and feelings about it.

- Be Present with your Being – allow yourself to be anchored in your powerful Now-consciousness.
- Positive Aspects – let yourself dwell on all that is going RIGHT with your physical system today.
- Appreciate! Appreciate! Appreciate! - allow yourself to tune into the cleansing, rejuvenating, and revitalizing power of the energy you physically experience in your state of appreciation.
- Release Resistance – before you withdraw from waking consciousness into your dream and sleep state, make it your intention to release whatever minor resistance you may have accumulated or created within your physical system on this day.

STREAM 17: YOUR BUILT-IN INDICATORS

The higher energies you physically translate as love, joy, and appreciation are not only feelings you experience in response to energy flowing freely through your physical apparatus, but are also indicators of the frequency field you are tuning into. Your feelings are constantly indicating to you what frequency domain and range you are tapping into in the instant you are experiencing these higher energies that you translate as love, joy, and appreciation.

The body-Universe reality that exists in the love-joy-bliss-appreciation grid is different from the body-Universe reality that exists in the disappointment-grid. They are different vibrational densities. They are different energetic platforms just as they are noticeably different states of being. Each frequency-range contains a version of your body and Universe, a version of your own self. Every grid or domain has its own frequency broadcast that you translate as the feelings of your physical experience. You are receiving constant feedback on energy flow and on what body-Universe reality you are tuning into, what reality you are materializing on your screen of experience.

Well-being is an experience of these higher energies. You, as Pure Consciousness, are in fact higher than even these higher energies. You translate the well-being of your True Nature as the general positive feelings you experience in your physical body. Who you really are, what you really are translates as energizing good feelings to your physical system. The more you train yourself to tune into the body-Universe reality that feels good, the more you attune yourself to these higher energies, the more you'll see your physical environment shift to materialize that good feeling body-Universe reality.

RECORD IN YOUR JOURNAL YOUR IMPRESSIONS OF THIS STREAM – *what is arising within you as you receive this particular stream? What are you experiencing mentally and physically as you read this stream? What questions or comments are arising in your awareness? Write your own translations of this stream down. Engage with the material to access your own wisdom and knowing.*

Daily Process
- Body Scan – first thing in the morning scan your physical body.
- Contemplate today's consciousness stream – allow yourself to visit today's thought and contemplate the idea presented to you. Come back to this idea frequently throughout your day. Write out your own translation of this stream, your initial impressions and feelings about it.
- Be Present with your Being – allow yourself to be anchored in your powerful Now-consciousness.
- Positive Aspects – let yourself dwell on all that is going RIGHT with your physical system today.
- Appreciate! Appreciate! Appreciate! - allow yourself to tune into the cleansing, rejuvenating, and revitalizing power of the energy you physically experience in your state of appreciation.

- Release Resistance – before you withdraw from waking consciousness into your dream and sleep state, make it your intention to release whatever minor resistance you may have accumulated or created within your physical system on this day.

STREAM 18: VIBRATIONAL INTERPRETATION

Take a look at your physical body in this instant. You are in the instant you observe your physical body actually really reading frequencies. What you perceive as your hands, your legs, what you look down and perceive as a body is an electrical translation of energy in motion. All of your senses, which themselves are frequency fields, are registering electronic data, or vibrational data, that your brain then reconstructs as a three-dimensional experience. The body you right now appear to experience only exists as a reconstruction of your nervous system.

Your brain-body apparatus acts as a quantum device that is decoding wave-patterns and reading them as the skin, legs, and various body parts you perceive. You are constantly interpreting and experiencing the translations of vibrational data like this. You are constantly registering electronic stimuli and translating them as physical experiences.

Everything you perceive is light and information, vibrational or electrical data. It isn't a solid and unchanging fixed reality that you are looking out upon. You are registering patterns of light-waves and the information you have been encoding onto your consciousness-matrix through the thoughts and beliefs you have continually accepted as valid.

As you change these thoughts and beliefs, as you tune into thoughts and beliefs of a different frequency range, you will begin to experience your physical body and its well-being completely differently. It is simple physics. The frequency you attune to as consciousness is the frequency you experience as a physical world. *As* within the consciousness that you are, so without in the world that appears external to you.

Daily Process
- Body Scan – first thing in the morning scan your physical body.
- Contemplate today's consciousness stream – allow yourself to visit today's thought and contemplate the idea presented to you. Come back to this idea frequently throughout your day. Write out your own translation of this stream, your initial impressions and feelings about it.
- Be Present with your Being – allow yourself to be anchored in your powerful Now-consciousness.
- Positive Aspects – let yourself dwell on all that is going RIGHT with your physical system today.
- Appreciate! Appreciate! Appreciate! - allow yourself to tune into the cleansing, rejuvenating, and revitalizing power of the energy you physically experience in your state of appreciation.
- Release Resistance – before you withdraw from waking consciousness into your dream and sleep state, make it your intention to release whatever minor resistance you may have accumulated or created within your physical system on this day.

MAKE a deliberate effort to record your response to this stream – what thoughts are arising as you engage with this stream of consciousness?

STREAM 19: SIMULTANEOUS REALITIES

The frequencies you generate within yourself through the thought-streams you tune into, accept, and empower determine what corresponding frequency domain, body-Universe reality, you experience as your physical and personal reality. There is no universe or physical reality that you perceive and participate in that is apart from the you-personality you have generated in this moment.

You are the information you experience at all times.

There is no "out there" separate and apart from the you-identity being generated in this instant. There is no outside world that is separate from the stream of consciousness you are flowing as in this moment. You are a unified stream with the world you appear to experience.

Whatever version of you that you tune into in this instant (i.e. the version of you that has always been healthy) resides in its own domain of experience. You are not a fixed single consciousness. All possible versions of you and their corresponding body-Universe reality, exist simultaneously, in the field of Infinite Information. There is no past or future, there is only the field of Now that contains all probable realities.

You and the body-Universe reality you experience are one simultaneous appearance. There is one singular flow that you experience as within yourself and outside yourself. It is all you. It is all the frequency that you are. Shift the frequency of your own being, shift the rate of vibration of your own consciousness, and you tune into the reality you want to experience. You do this by tuning into thoughts in harmony with the body-Universe reality you desire. You are the frequency dial you adjust to experience the reality you prefer.

Be the frequency you wish to experience. Be the well-being you wish to experience. Be the vibration you wish to see reflected in your physical system and world.

QUESTIONS TO ANSWER IN YOUR JOURNAL:

What is the feel of your ideal body-Universe reality?

What is the moment to moment feeling of your perfect body-Universe reality?

What thoughts can you focus on to feel these feelings now?

If you were to right now view your world from the state of already experiencing your most ideal body-Universe reality, what details would you be noticing?

If all that was here right now all around you, in every direction was your already living in your most ideal body-Universe reality, what changes?

What are you experiencing as you engage with these questions?

Daily Process

- Body Scan – first thing in the morning scan your physical body.
- Contemplate today's consciousness stream – allow yourself to visit today's thought and contemplate the idea presented to you. Come back to this idea frequently throughout your

day. Write out your own translation of this stream, your initial impressions and feelings about it.

- Be Present with your Being – allow yourself to be anchored in your powerful Now-consciousness.
- Positive Aspects – let yourself dwell on all that is going RIGHT with your physical system today.
- Appreciate! Appreciate! Appreciate! - allow yourself to tune into the cleansing, rejuvenating, and revitalizing power of the energy you physically experience in your state of appreciation.
- Release Resistance – before you withdraw from waking consciousness into your dream and sleep state, make it your intention to release whatever minor resistance you may have accumulated or created within your physical system on this day.

STREAM 20: YOUR NATURE IS TO THRIVE

Unlimited thinking, thoughts of limitless possibilities, resonate at a high frequency. Absolute well-being and limitless possibilities are your natural expansive states of being. You are by nature a consciousness stream of absolute well-being and limitless potential. There is nothing that you cannot bring into your world, for yours is a reality of endless possibilities. There is no experience you cannot bring into your experience, for yours is a world of infinite and never-ending potentialities. You are unlimited in every sense of the world.

The more you allow yourself to tune out of the limiting beliefs you have picked up in the course of your physical focus, the more you break free from mass consciousness and the information offered to you about what's true for your individual physical body, the more easily you will naturally materialize and externalize your infinite miraculous nature and power to be in a state of unwavering wellness. Wellness of body, wellness of mind, wellness of heart, wellness of circumstances and situations are all natural for you in your true core state of being.

You are not here to materialize what all others have materialized. You are not here to recreate the misunderstandings of others into your experience. You are not here to mimic and parrot the limited stories of those before you. You are here to reveal the limitless nature of who and what you really are. Your very nature is to thrive, expand, and reveal your own limitlessness.

Daily Process
- Body Scan – first thing in the morning scan your physical body.
- Contemplate today's consciousness stream – allow yourself to visit today's thought and contemplate the idea presented to you. Come back to this idea frequently throughout your day. Write out your own translation of this stream, your initial impressions and feelings about it.
- Be Present with your Being – allow yourself to be anchored in your powerful Now-consciousness.
- Positive Aspects – let yourself dwell on all that is going RIGHT with your physical system today.
- Appreciate! Appreciate! Appreciate! - allow yourself to tune into the cleansing, rejuvenating, and revitalizing power of the energy you physically experience in your state of appreciation.
- Release Resistance – before you withdraw from waking consciousness into your dream and sleep state, make it your intention to release whatever minor resistance you may have accumulated or created within your physical system on this day.

STREAM 21: TUNING INTO THE REAL YOU

Every frequency domain you tune into and participate in offers you information to install into your consciousness-matrix, the blueprint of your physical body and personal reality. You are constantly being offered information on what can or cannot happen to the physical body. You are not offered truth. You are offered information. What validates any information, what makes any information true is your acceptance of it. There are no truths in this reality, there are only information streams. And you have choice in what information streams, what programs you integrate into your personal reality. The more you tune into your ability to consciously choose your preferred body-Universe reality, the more you break free from the limited ideas you are offered to experience the body-Universe reality you desire to experience.

You are not a limited physical being in a hard mass of an unchanging physical body and Universe. You are not what a world blind and asleep says you are. You are not an extension of limitedness and frailty. You are an expression of a boundless flawless intelligence. You are pure light and information shifting in wave-like domains of experience. You are Liquid Consciousness participating in the illusion of time, space, and solidity. You are an extension, an exact duplicate, of the Infinite Intelligence that brings intricate Universes into being. You are more space than you are physical malleable matter, and more free and subtle than even thoughts vibrating at the highest frequencies. You are higher than even the highest energies. You are higher than even the highest ideas.

You are much more than concepts and words can point to. Tune in to the Real You.

QUESTION TO ANSWER IN YOUR JOURNAL:
Where are you allowing limited ideas, low frequency information to influence your body-Universe experience?

Daily Process
- Body Scan – first thing in the morning scan your physical body.
- Contemplate today's consciousness stream – allow yourself to visit today's thought and contemplate the idea presented to you. Come back to this idea frequently throughout your day. Write out your own translation of this stream, your initial impressions and feelings about it.
- Be Present with your Being – allow yourself to be anchored in your powerful Now-consciousness.
- Positive Aspects – let yourself dwell on all that is going RIGHT with your physical system today.
- Appreciate! Appreciate! Appreciate! - allow yourself to tune into the cleansing, rejuvenating, and revitalizing power of the energy you physically experience in your state of appreciation.
- Release Resistance – before you withdraw from waking consciousness into your dream and sleep state, make it your intention to release whatever minor resistance you may have accumulated or created within your physical system on this day.

STREAM 22: YOUR NEW BEGINNING

Past and future do not exist. Whatever materialized as your yesterday is a potential signal out of an infinite many that you are tuning into in this instant of pure power. Memories, like all else that you experience, are frequency patterns you are tuning into. Yesterday is a potential pattern of information you are accessing Now. Tomorrow is a potential signal you are accessing Now. You can at any point recede into your Singularity, the dimension you experience and translate as the Stillness within yourself, and re-emerge into the frequency domain and body-Universe reality you prefer to experience. Your preferred reality is only a thought-stream away.

Nothing is done or complete. No appearing condition is a final sentence. No diagnosis is an only possibility. Everything, every aspect of your physical experience, is a potential reality you are accessing in this very instant, and you can easily tune out of it and into something else, into an alternate stream of information. Now is all there is, and right Now offers you a clean slate, a fresh start, a new beginning to step into the reality you prefer.

If you can release the version of yesterday you experienced and tune into your preferred yesterday, you will shift the parallel and simultaneous stream of reality you are experiencing as your physical body and life. Remember, everything is a stream of information you are accessing, and there is no limit to what information stream you tune into. If you can release your attachment to the story of your yesterday and your limited projections of tomorrow, you can free yourself to tune into the reality of your ever-present and unfailing absolute well-being.

Daily Process
- Body Scan – first thing in the morning scan your physical body.
- Contemplate today's consciousness stream – allow yourself to visit today's thought and contemplate the idea presented to you. Come back to this idea frequently throughout your day. Write out your own translation of this stream, your initial impressions and feelings about it.
- Be Present with your Being – allow yourself to be anchored in your powerful Now-consciousness.
- Positive Aspects – let yourself dwell on all that is going RIGHT with your physical system today.
- Appreciate! Appreciate! Appreciate! - allow yourself to tune into the cleansing, rejuvenating, and revitalizing power of the energy you physically experience in your state of appreciation.
- Release Resistance – before you withdraw from waking consciousness into your dream and sleep state, make it your intention to release whatever minor resistance you may have accumulated or created within your physical system on this day.

STREAM 23: NEVER CEASE CHOOSING YOUR PREFERRED REALITY

There is no limit to what frequency domain you can tune into in each one of your moments. There is no limit to how many times you choose to tune into the frequency domain of absolute well-being. The only place is Here and the only time is Now, so the only question is what vibrational field are you choosing to tune into in this moment?

Whatever condition appeared in your experience of yesterday is information you are choosing to include in your experience of today. Today is not a continuation of a perceived yesterday. You can in this moment tune into the simultaneous reality in which no such condition ever existed. Take a moment to see how you are accessing the information stream of your yesterday. *Where is yesterday right now? Can you locate it without turning to thought-patterns, recollections, images your mind brings up?*

Yesterday is only a thought-pattern you are tuning into in this moment. It isn't here. You are choosing to tune into it. Right here and right now is your new beginning, a beginning in which you can choose what you create as your total physical experience. Every Now moment offers you a chance to tune again and again into your preferred reality. What appeared to happen yesterday isn't happening right now, unless you are tuning into the thought-pattern that contradicts this.

Even if it appears to you that you seem to tune in and out of your preferred reality, Now offers you a chance to choose again.

Daily Process
- Body Scan – first thing in the morning scan your physical body.
- Contemplate today's consciousness stream – allow yourself to visit today's thought and contemplate the idea presented to you. Come back to this idea frequently throughout your day. Write out your own translation of this stream, your initial impressions and feelings about it.
- Be Present with your Being – allow yourself to be anchored in your powerful Now-consciousness.
- Positive Aspects – let yourself dwell on all that is going RIGHT with your physical system today.
- Appreciate! Appreciate! Appreciate! – allow yourself to tune into the cleansing, rejuvenating, and revitalizing power of the energy you physically experience in your state of appreciation.
- Release Resistance – before you withdraw from waking consciousness into your dream and sleep state, make it your intention to release whatever minor resistance you may have accumulated or created within your physical system on this day.

STREAM 24: TUNING INTO YOUR ALIGNED BODY

You cannot tune into the thought-pattern, the vibration, of a perfectly functioning physical body at the same time that you tune into a body filled with discomfort. They are different thought-streams giving you access to different realities. They are from different vibrational domains. They are different energy streams.

Both streams are available to you in this instant. It merely requires a shift in what thought-streams you tune into for you to experience the reality of these simultaneous thought-streams. You can choose to tune into all the moments in which you experienced your physical body in perfect form, in perfect health, thriving and working flawlessly. You can just as easily choose to conjure up images of well-being as you do images of the absence of well-being. And you can let your ability to deliberately direct your attention to focus on the images, to tune into the signals, that represent the reality you desire to experience.

Allow yourself to tune into these thought-streams and images of thriving, being well, feeling vigorous, being vibrant, being and feeling lively. For as you do, you release all resistance to experiencing the reality of your aligned body. Whatever resistance you experience as symptoms dissolves the moment you shift your focus and attention toward images and thought-streams that return the flow of energy in and through your physical system to normal.

Today's Processes
- Body Scan – first thing in the morning scan your

physical body.
- Contemplate today's consciousness stream – allow yourself to visit today's thought and contemplate the idea presented to you. Come back to this idea frequently throughout your day. Write out your own translation of this stream, your initial impressions and feelings about it.
- Be Present with your Being – allow yourself to be anchored in your powerful Now-consciousness.
- Positive Aspects – let yourself dwell on all that is going RIGHT with your physical system today.
- Appreciate! Appreciate! Appreciate! - allow yourself to tune into the cleansing, rejuvenating, and revitalizing power of the energy you physically experience in your state of appreciation.
- Release Resistance – before you withdraw from waking consciousness into your dream and sleep state, make it your intention to release whatever minor resistance you may have accumulated or created within your physical system on this day.

STREAM 25: YOUR POWER OF FOCUS

The feeling tones you experience are constantly indicating to you the vibrational domain you are tuning into. And the frequency, or feeling, you generate within yourself on any topic in this moment determines what frames of experience appear as your next moment, and the moment after that.

You have the power to generate any feeling within yourself in this moment through the power of your focus regardless of what circumstances or conditions you are facing. Circumstances are secondary. The primary factor is the frequency of your own being, and you have absolute power over that. Consciousness, the state of being you possess in any given moment is the sole cause of what shows up in your world. You have the absolute power to choose the essence of what you will experience as your upcoming segments, as you have the ability to be vibrating at any frequency in this moment.

Where you appear to be right now is a passing vibrational indicator revealing to you the balance of your thoughts, the thoughts and beliefs you have been practicing up until now. What appears in this moment is transient, it is passing. And its duration is only determined by how you are continuing to empower it. What is appearing as your reality in this instant can dissolve, shift, or transform in the blink of an eye.

If you recognize that your manifested world is just a vibrational indicator, that it is only a mirror reflecting to you where you have been vibrating, and begin to tune into higher-frequency thought-patterns, better feeling thoughts, then its duration is shortened.

Allow yourself to let go of holding the manifested world to be more than it is. Allow yourself to experience the malleability of your world. Allow yourself to experience your ability to instantly shift out of any appearance. You can.

Daily Process
- Body Scan – first thing in the morning scan your physical body.
- Contemplate today's consciousness stream – allow yourself to visit today's thought and contemplate the idea presented to you. Come back to this idea frequently throughout your day. Write out your own translation of this stream, your initial impressions and feelings about it.
- Be Present with your Being – allow yourself to be anchored in your powerful Now-consciousness.
- Positive Aspects – let yourself dwell on all that is going RIGHT with your physical system today.
- Appreciate! Appreciate! Appreciate! - allow yourself to tune into the cleansing, rejuvenating, and revitalizing power of the energy you physically experience in your state of appreciation.
- Release Resistance – before you withdraw from waking consciousness into your dream and sleep state, make it your intention to release whatever minor resistance you may have accumulated or created within your physical system on this day.

STREAM 26: A HIGH-FREQUENCY THOUGHT IS A NATURAL REMEDY

The various remedies you turn to are the permission slips you give to yourself to experience your natural well-being. Pay attention to the turnaround in your thoughts when you take your medicines, supplements, or treatments. Your unquestioning belief that these remedies will work automatically has you tuning into thoughts vibrating at a higher frequency.

Your remedies are useful to you. There is no need to negate their value for they too are consciousness, streams of information.

What this is pointing you toward is the self-awareness in what begins to happen to you internally, in the balance of your thoughts and expectations.

As you take your medicines, you naturally begin to release resistant thought-patterns and allow yourself to tune into your preferred body-Universe reality. You naturally begin to expect wellness. You naturally begin to feel better about the condition you find yourself in. You naturally begin to feel hopeful and embrace the possibility of wellness once again. Notice the often immediate turnaround in your vibration, in your inner-tone or frequency, when you reach for relief in the various treatments available to you.

With this recognition you can begin to tune into thoughts vibrating at higher frequencies even prior to reaching for physical remedies, at the onset of symptoms or mild discomforts. Thoughts vibrating at higher frequencies always translate into an experience of well-being in all facets of your physical life. You can train yourself to stabilize in a vibrational field where such thoughts are dominant and so can experience how truly self-sufficient you have been designed to be.

You are perfectly designed to thrive at all times!

Daily Process
- Body Scan – first thing in the morning scan your physical body.
- Contemplate today's consciousness stream – allow yourself to visit today's thought and contemplate the idea presented to you. Come back to this idea frequently throughout your day. Write out your own translation of this stream, your initial impressions and feelings about it.
- Be Present with your Being – allow yourself to be anchored in your powerful Now-consciousness.
- Positive Aspects – let yourself dwell on all that is going RIGHT with your physical system today.
- Appreciate! Appreciate! Appreciate! - allow yourself to tune into the cleansing, rejuvenating, and revitalizing power of the energy you physically experience in your state of appreciation.
- Release Resistance – before you withdraw from waking consciousness into your dream and sleep state, make it your intention to release whatever minor resistance you may have accumulated or created within your physical system on this day.

STREAM 27: THE DISAPPEARANCE OF RESISTANT PATTERNS

There is not a single condition that appears that is not an indicator of resistance, of you remaining focused in a vibrational domain that is dense with resistant thought-streams. Disease is always revealing to you the effect of the resistant thought-streams, all those little bothers and frustrations, that you tune into and keep active in your personal energy field. Whatever resistant pattern you create in your energy field remains unless you release it. All disease is the cumulative effect of resistant thought patterns. All disease is indicating to you what the vibrational frequency of the balance of your thoughts, the thought-patterns you frequently tune into, is. There are no exceptions.

There are no diseases that appear for another reason. There are no discomforts or maladies that appear in the absence of resistance. Resistance is always the cause of unwanted manifestations. It is always a play of energy and balance. It is always an indication of energy flow. The reason is always about how you have allowed or dis-allowed the high-frequency energy, life force, to flow through your physical system. Every single time, that is what it's all about.

And the form the resistance takes, the type of condition that appears to develop, is in line with what you believe you can develop or manifest in your physical body. Everything is a translation of vibrational patterns, and so the way the resistance translates within your physical reality is by appearing to be some disease you have taken to be real.

You can see through this illusion and recognize that no matter the form of the appearing disease, it is only your translation of the resistance you have built up. It isn't anything else. It is a vibrational translation, a reading of frequencies like all other things. So as you release this resistance by tuning into higher-frequency thoughts, better feeling thoughts, this energy pattern or pattern of resistance will cease appearing in your physical reality. Without question.

Daily Process
- Body Scan – first thing in the morning scan your physical body.
- Contemplate today's consciousness stream – allow yourself to visit today's thought and contemplate the idea presented to you. Come back to this idea frequently throughout your day. Write out your own translation of this stream, your initial impressions and feelings about it.
- Be Present with your Being – allow yourself to be anchored in your powerful Now-consciousness.
- Positive Aspects – let yourself dwell on all that is going RIGHT with your physical system today.
- Appreciate! Appreciate! Appreciate! - allow yourself to tune into the cleansing, rejuvenating, and revitalizing power of the energy you physically experience in your state of appreciation.
- Release Resistance – before you withdraw from waking consciousness into your dream and sleep state, make it your intention to release whatever

minor resistance you may have accumulated or created within your physical system on this day.

STREAM 28: THE STORY YOU TELL

In each moment you are committing to the reality you are going to participate in. Every personal story you tell in your mind and express, every train of thought you allow to remain active within yourself, focuses your physical reality and experience to look and feel a certain way. It is your choice of focus in this moment, the story you are keeping active in your mind of what's valid and real for you, that determines which body-Universe reality you are going to experience. The story you activate and tell about your world, about your body, about your reality and yourself, in this moment is everything.

What story are you telling?

Daily Process
- Body Scan – first thing in the morning scan your physical body.
- Contemplate today's consciousness stream – allow yourself to visit today's thought and contemplate the idea presented to you. Come back to this idea frequently throughout your day. Write out your own translation of this stream, your initial impressions and feelings about it.
- Be Present with your Being – allow yourself to be anchored in your powerful Now-consciousness.
- Positive Aspects – let yourself dwell on all that is going RIGHT with your physical system today.
- Appreciate! Appreciate! Appreciate! - allow

yourself to tune into the cleansing, rejuvenating, and revitalizing power of the energy you physically experience in your state of appreciation.

- Release Resistance – before you withdraw from waking consciousness into your dream and sleep state, make it your intention to release whatever minor resistance you may have accumulated or created within your physical system on this day.

STREAM 29: ENERGY BODY

You have the ability to perceive every layer of your being as energy, as a frequency field, as pure light.
Begin this exercise at the bottom of your feet and work your way up to the top of your head. As you run your awareness up the body, focus on each body part. Allow yourself to recognize and experience it as energy, as pure light. Hold your attention on each body part and expand that perception. Deepen your perception of being an energy system. See each part of your physical body as actually being particles flickering in and out of visibility. See each part of the body as being mostly made up of empty space. See light flooding trillions of energy pathways all throughout the body.
Let go of the perception of physical solid parts. Let go of the perception of extremities and organs, bones and muscles, vessels and cells. Instead of seeing toes, legs, fingers, eyes, ears, or hair, allow yourself to see and experience each of these areas as light, as tiny vibrating particles. See yourself immersed in an ocean of light. Allow yourself to experience the expansiveness, the openness, the weightlessness of this lens.

Daily Process
- Body Scan – first thing in the morning scan your physical body.
- Contemplate today's consciousness stream – allow yourself to visit today's thought and contemplate the idea presented to you. Come back to this idea frequently throughout your

day. Write out your own translation of this stream, your initial impressions and feelings about it.

- Be Present with your Being – allow yourself to be anchored in your powerful Now-consciousness.
- Positive Aspects – let yourself dwell on all that is going RIGHT with your physical system today.
- Appreciate! Appreciate! Appreciate! – allow yourself to tune into the cleansing, rejuvenating, and revitalizing power of the energy you physically experience in your state of appreciation.
- Release Resistance – before you withdraw from waking consciousness into your dream and sleep state, make it your intention to release whatever minor resistance you may have accumulated or created within your physical system on this day.

STREAM 30: STEPPING INTO VIBRATIONAL HARMONY WITH PREFERRED REALITY

The easiest way to tune into and participate in your preferred body-Universe reality is to align yourself to the highest frequencies of your personal reality, to the things that excite, inspire, and uplift you. Stay tuned into and continue to participate in the activities, the conversations, the gatherings, that line you up to these higher frequencies you translate as joy, love, appreciation, or excitement.

Consciously and deliberately align yourself to these energies by focusing on thought-streams that generate these higher frequencies within you. Appreciate more. Love more. Step into the stream of joy more. Be excited more. Feel passion more. Think about the things that inspire you. Focus on the things, the stories, the people, that uplift you. Surround yourself with higher vibrations.

The energies you translate as good feelings, the aspects of your reality that evoke good feelings within you, are always indicating to you that you in these instances are open and flowing energy without restriction. They are telling you that you are tuned into and in harmony with your most preferred body-Universe reality.

Daily Process
- Body Scan – first thing in the morning scan your physical body.
- Contemplate today's consciousness stream – allow yourself to visit today's thought and contemplate the idea presented to you. Come

back to this idea frequently throughout your day. Write out your own translation of this stream, your initial impressions and feelings about it.

- Be Present with your Being – allow yourself to be anchored in your powerful Now-consciousness.
- Positive Aspects – let yourself dwell on all that is going RIGHT with your physical system today.
- Appreciate! Appreciate! Appreciate! - allow yourself to tune into the cleansing, rejuvenating, and revitalizing power of the energy you physically experience in your state of appreciation.
- Release Resistance – before you withdraw from waking consciousness into your dream and sleep state, make it your intention to release whatever minor resistance you may have accumulated or created within your physical system on this day.

STREAM 31: YOU ARE THE ULTIMATE AUTHORITY

Your experience of absolute well-being has a direct correlation to your decision to put your focus on the thoughts, information, and events that evoke good feelings within you. Good feelings are always indicating to you the flow of pure energy through your physical apparatus. Good feelings are indicators of your inevitable well-being. It is the power of your own focus, where you allow your attention to dwell, that can lift you out of the resistant patterns you experience as all disease and discomfort.

The flow of unlimited energy is available to you in this instant, and it is the effort you make within yourself to shift what you focus on and express that takes you into that flow and preferred experience. You are the ultimate authority on where you put your attention and what vibrations you allow to influence your state of well-being. You are the only authority on what you choose to accept and integrate into your outlook, your vibration lens of perception.

You are absolutely the sole author of all that you make manifest in and as your body-Universe reality. Own your power!

Daily Process
- Body Scan – first thing in the morning scan your physical body.
- Contemplate today's consciousness stream – allow yourself to visit today's thought and contemplate the idea presented to you. Come

back to this idea frequently throughout your day. Write out your own translation of this stream, your initial impressions and feelings about it.
- Be Present with your Being – allow yourself to be anchored in your powerful Now-consciousness.
- Positive Aspects – let yourself dwell on all that is going RIGHT with your physical system today.
- Appreciate! Appreciate! Appreciate! - allow yourself to tune into the cleansing, rejuvenating, and revitalizing power of the energy you physically experience in your state of appreciation.
- Release Resistance – before you withdraw from waking consciousness into your dream and sleep state, make it your intention to release whatever minor resistance you may have accumulated or created within your physical system on this day.

STREAM 32: YOUR PHYSICAL BODY IS MAGNIFICENT

Your physical body, your physical apparatus is designed to thrive. It is designed to replenish itself. It is designed to repair itself. Your physical body knows exactly what it needs to do and has quantum access to the infinite field of pure potential. It has immediate access to the endless reservoir of pure energy that constructs Universes. It is naturally inclined to be a harmonious, adaptable, and extraordinary system able to allow you to experience this seemingly physical Universe with effortless ease.

Your body is one hundred percent energy, pure vibration. It is pure power. It is pure electricity. It is pure intelligence. It is made of the same miraculous substance that creates vast and complex Universes. Its intelligence is beyond anything your conscious mind can comprehend even with all of your advanced understanding and technology.

And as you appreciate, love, and acknowledge the superiority of your own physical apparatus, its design, and miraculous potential, you will train yourself into allowing your physical body's natural ability to be the thriving, harmonious, resilient, magnificent system it is designed to be.

Daily Process
- Body Scan – first thing in the morning scan your physical body.
- Contemplate today's consciousness stream – allow yourself to visit today's thought and contemplate the idea presented to you. Come

back to this idea frequently throughout your day. Write out your own translation of this stream, your initial impressions and feelings about it.
- Be Present with your Being – allow yourself to be anchored in your powerful Now-consciousness.
- Positive Aspects – let yourself dwell on all that is going RIGHT with your physical system today.
- Appreciate! Appreciate! Appreciate! – allow yourself to tune into the cleansing, rejuvenating, and revitalizing power of the energy you physically experience in your state of appreciation.
- Release Resistance – before you withdraw from waking consciousness into your dream and sleep state, make it your intention to release whatever minor resistance you may have accumulated or created within your physical system on this day.

STREAM 33: CONSCIOUSNESS IS THE ONLY POWER

The only power in your experience is Consciousness. Consciousness is the sole power, the sole author, and the single Source of all that appears in your reality. There has never been any other power. There has never been any other authority. All the power has always resided in your being. And so it is by changing your own consciousness that you change the scenery of your waking world. It is by changing the speed of vibration of your own being, that you give yourself access to more desirable experiences. There is no "out there" to combat, to resist, or to struggle against. Let your own consciousness be central to your experience.

If you can allow your own consciousness to be the sole cause of all that comes into your world, only then do you give yourself the full power to change or transform whatever comes. How empowered you are in your reality is entirely up to you. How much power you experience to change, transform, or shift anything that arises in your experiences, is entirely up to you.

You are consciousness, and so you are the power in your reality, you are the power in this moment, you are the power in your world.

Daily Process
- Body Scan – first thing in the morning scan your physical body.
- Contemplate today's consciousness stream – allow yourself to visit today's thought and contemplate the idea presented to you. Come

back to this idea frequently throughout your day. Write out your own translation of this stream, your initial impressions and feelings about it.
- Be Present with your Being – allow yourself to be anchored in your powerful Now-consciousness.
- Positive Aspects – let yourself dwell on all that is going RIGHT with your physical system today.
- Appreciate! Appreciate! Appreciate! - allow yourself to tune into the cleansing, rejuvenating, and revitalizing power of the energy you physically experience in your state of appreciation.
- Release Resistance – before you withdraw from waking consciousness into your dream and sleep state, make it your intention to release whatever minor resistance you may have accumulated or created within your physical system on this day.

STREAM 34: HABITUATING HIGHER-FREQUENCY THOUGHT STREAMS

The more you consider just exactly how your body works the more you will shake off the false notion that you are made of flesh and bones. Even the visible layer of your physical body is energy vibrating at a specific frequency. Everything about you is energy vibrating at various frequencies. You are pure light and information vibrating in accord to the frequencies you have calibrated yourself to.

The beliefs you hold are practiced patterns of vibration – these too are energy patterns. And it is these beliefs, which vibrate at a higher frequency than the denser seemingly material aspect of your body, that regulate and direct the conditions that materialize in your body-Universe reality. Your world flowers out of the vibrations you practice. Your reality emerges out of the thought-feeling frequencies you constantly attune yourself to and emanate out of your consciousness-matrix.

Every thought you think vibrates, and every thought you think repeatedly becomes part of your template of experience, it becomes a belief, a well-rehearsed vibration. The more you deliberately tune into the higher frequency thought-streams, the more these thought-streams habituate and become dominant. With practice you can stabilize in your preferred frequency-range of experience. You can align and harmonize yourself to a different range of frequencies. Remember, it is when you change the frequency of your own consciousness-matrix that you change the structure and appearance of your waking world.

Daily Process

- Body Scan – first thing in the morning scan your physical body.
- Contemplate today's consciousness stream – allow yourself to visit today's thought and contemplate the idea presented to you. Come back to this idea frequently throughout your day. Write out your own translation of this stream, your initial impressions and feelings about it.
- Be Present with your Being – allow yourself to be anchored in your powerful Now-consciousness.
- Positive Aspects – let yourself dwell on all that is going RIGHT with your physical system today.
- Appreciate! Appreciate! Appreciate! – allow yourself to tune into the cleansing, rejuvenating, and revitalizing power of the energy you physically experience in your state of appreciation.
- Release Resistance – before you withdraw from waking consciousness into your dream and sleep state, make it your intention to release whatever minor resistance you may have accumulated or created within your physical system on this day.

STREAM 35: THOUGHT IS THE FIRST STEP

You cannot tune into your preferred body-Universe reality while staying focused on your current reality, while continuing to flow your energy into your current stream of thoughts. You must be willing to look past the temporary picture on your screen of experience and let go of the active thoughts within you, in this instant.

Recognize what appears in this instant for what it is and immediately shift your attention and focus onto the thought-streams, the pattern of thinking that will allow you to tune into the frequency domain of your preferred body-Universe reality. What alters your reality begins with the thought-streams and corresponding emotional indicators you generate within your own consciousness.

Thought is always the first step you take, everything else is secondary. You have the innate ability to direct your thoughts only to go in the direction of your preferred experience.

Daily Process
- Body Scan – first thing in the morning scan your physical body.
- Contemplate today's consciousness stream – allow yourself to visit today's thought and contemplate the idea presented to you. Come back to this idea frequently throughout your day. Write out your own translation of this stream, your initial impressions and feelings about it.
- Be Present with your Being – allow yourself to

be anchored in your powerful Now-consciousness.

- Positive Aspects – let yourself dwell on all that is going RIGHT with your physical system today.
- Appreciate! Appreciate! Appreciate! – allow yourself to tune into the cleansing, rejuvenating, and revitalizing power of the energy you physically experience in your state of appreciation.
- Release Resistance – before you withdraw from waking consciousness into your dream and sleep state, make it your intention to release whatever minor resistance you may have accumulated or created within your physical system on this day.

STREAM 36: EXPANDING YOUR BELIEF PARAMETERS

You can deliberately use the regulating and directing power of your beliefs to your benefit by creating new beliefs, by installing new patterns of energy that correspond to the body-Universe reality you want to experience. If your desire is to experience absolute physical well-being, then you must install the beliefs, the energy patterns, that will allow for your natural inclination toward thriving and well-being to manifest.

Your reality cannot materialize outside of your belief parameters, the thoughts you have practiced and continue to practice. The apparent facts of your holographic reality, are only beliefs you have practiced and created a consensus around. You can at any point choose to break free of these agreed upon belief boundaries on what your physical body can be, do, and become.

Anything outside of your belief boundaries, any evidence or stream of information that can show you what absolute physical well-being looks like will be invisible to you for such evidence is outside of your frequency range. The way to come into range is to consciously and deliberately tune yourself into the thought-streams that will allow you to experience the absolute physical well-being natural to you. The more you come into harmony with higher frequency thought-streams, the more you release your practiced resistance to your natural and absolute well-being.

Daily Process

- Body Scan – first thing in the morning scan your physical body.
- Contemplate today's consciousness stream – allow yourself to visit today's thought and contemplate the idea presented to you. Come back to this idea frequently throughout your day. Write out your own translation of this stream, your initial impressions and feelings about it.
- Be Present with your Being – allow yourself to be anchored in your powerful Now-consciousness.
- Positive Aspects – let yourself dwell on all that is going RIGHT with your physical system today.
- Appreciate! Appreciate! Appreciate! - allow yourself to tune into the cleansing, rejuvenating, and revitalizing power of the energy you physically experience in your state of appreciation.
- Release Resistance – before you withdraw from waking consciousness into your dream and sleep state, make it your intention to release whatever minor resistance you may have accumulated or created within your physical system on this day.

STREAM 37: YOU ARE THE POWER OF YOUR PERSONAL REALITY

You cannot believe in sickness and disease, and continually manifest physical well-being. You cannot believe in vulnerability and manifest immunity. Your beliefs open you up to the information and evidence of their own content.

Beliefs are by nature self-perpetuating intelligent mechanisms that will continue to validate themselves before your eyes. Think differently, believe differently, and all the conditions you once believed were real will dissolve before you.

You are the only power keeping the information streams that make themselves known to you visible. You are the only power keeping them alive. You are the only author of your personal reality. What you know comes into being. What you believe comes into being. What you validate as true will manifest in your experience. You are infallible in your own personal reality as all things conspire to conform and give evidence to what you hold to be real and true. Just as you are what makes all experiences true and valid for your personal reality, you are what can make them equally untrue.

Daily Process
- Body Scan – first thing in the morning scan your physical body.
- Contemplate today's consciousness stream – allow yourself to visit today's thought and contemplate the idea presented to you. Come back to this idea frequently throughout your

day. Write out your own translation of this stream, your initial impressions and feelings about it.

- Be Present with your Being – allow yourself to be anchored in your powerful Now-consciousness.
- Positive Aspects – let yourself dwell on all that is going RIGHT with your physical system today.
- Appreciate! Appreciate! Appreciate! - allow yourself to tune into the cleansing, rejuvenating, and revitalizing power of the energy you physically experience in your state of appreciation.
- Release Resistance – before you withdraw from waking consciousness into your dream and sleep state, make it your intention to release whatever minor resistance you may have accumulated or created within your physical system on this day.

STREAM 38: THE NATURE OF DIS-EASE

Every disease ever known or yet to be discovered is your interpretation or translation of resistance. Resistance is the cause and resistance is the manifestation. You give this translation of resistance various names, classes, and definitions, but at the root of all that appears as illness or disease to you, is resistance.

There is no such thing as a disease that appears for no reason. There is no such thing as a virus that appears for no reason. There is no such thing as an illness that appears for no reason. All of it is your interpretation of resistance. All of it is vibrational data, energetic feedback. You have classified and given reality to resistant patterns of thought as independent entities in your physical universe, but they are not what they appear to be. Nothing is as it appears to be and nothing is what you have thought it to be.

Everything that is visible to you is your interpretation of wave-patterns. Everything that appears as your physical world is your translation of light and information, of frequency fields. You are a vibrational interpreter, an energetic transmitter and receiver of information. You are an electric being participating in the illusion of physical reality. There is not a single moment in which you are not translating patterns of energy, registering electrical stimuli and perceiving a three-dimensional world out of these patterns of light.

Daily Process
- Body Scan – first thing in the morning scan your

physical body.

- Contemplate today's consciousness stream – allow yourself to visit today's thought and contemplate the idea presented to you. Come back to this idea frequently throughout your day. Write out your own translation of this stream, your initial impressions and feelings about it.
- Be Present with your Being – allow yourself to be anchored in your powerful Now-consciousness.
- Positive Aspects – let yourself dwell on all that is going RIGHT with your physical system today.
- Appreciate! Appreciate! Appreciate! - allow yourself to tune into the cleansing, rejuvenating, and revitalizing power of the energy you physically experience in your state of appreciation.
- Release Resistance – before you withdraw from waking consciousness into your dream and sleep state, make it your intention to release whatever minor resistance you may have accumulated or created within your physical system on this day.

STREAM 39: THE POWER OF STILLNESS

The energy stream you translate as Stillness is available to you in this immediate instant. This immediate instant, the only creative point where the physical universe and the non-physical Source, Consciousness, meet offers you an endless new beginning. Right now is your new beginning.

You can step out of the illusion of time and linear perception into this ever-present space of ease and lightness. You can withdraw from the entire thought-stream you have been tuning into to rest in this state that your physical body can only translate as Stillness.

Bringing all of your awareness into your Still Center instantly clears and cleanses the octaves of your energy field. One of the fastest ways to release resistance immediately, to release the blockages from the various layers of your Being is to Be Still and allow this high frequency you translate as Stillness to pulse through every layer of your energetic structure and system. From Here you can then more easily restart your focus in the direction of your preferred reality.

Daily Process
- Body Scan – first thing in the morning scan your physical body.
- Contemplate today's consciousness stream – allow yourself to visit today's thought and contemplate the idea presented to you. Come back to this idea frequently throughout your day. Write out your own translation of this stream, your initial impressions and feelings

about it.

- Be Present with your Being – allow yourself to be anchored in your powerful Now-consciousness.
- Positive Aspects – let yourself dwell on all that is going RIGHT with your physical system today.
- Appreciate! Appreciate! Appreciate! - allow yourself to tune into the cleansing, rejuvenating, and revitalizing power of the energy you physically experience in your state of appreciation.
- Release Resistance – before you withdraw from waking consciousness into your dream and sleep state, make it your intention to release whatever minor resistance you may have accumulated or created within your physical system on this day.

STREAM 40: CHOOSING WELL-BEING FROM MOMENT-TO-MOMENT

There is no manifestation of resistance that comes instantaneously as a disease or discomfort. It is the resistance you have built up over time that manifests as what you translate or interpret as disease and illness. It is the little worries, frustrations, and general feelings of fear and insecurity that pinch off the flow of universal power to the point that over time the pattern of resistance begins to appear as disease and degeneration.

It is in the management of your day to day vibration, the thought-streams and frequency domains you attune yourself to and harmonize with that determine what will show up in and as your physical reality. Your well-being is a moment-to-moment choice of focus. Your power to deliberately choose where your attention goes, your power to deliberately become conscious of and choose what you are focusing on makes you the ultimate decider, the ultimate authority, of what materializes in and as your body-Universe reality.

Daily Process

- Body Scan – first thing in the morning scan your physical body.
- Contemplate today's consciousness stream – allow yourself to visit today's thought and contemplate the idea presented to you. Come back to this idea frequently throughout your day. Write out your own translation of this stream, your initial impressions and feelings

about it.

- Be Present with your Being – allow yourself to be anchored in your powerful Now-consciousness.
- Positive Aspects – let yourself dwell on all that is going RIGHT with your physical system today.
- Appreciate! Appreciate! Appreciate! - allow yourself to tune into the cleansing, rejuvenating, and revitalizing power of the energy you physically experience in your state of appreciation.
- Release Resistance – before you withdraw from waking consciousness into your dream and sleep state, make it your intention to release whatever minor resistance you may have accumulated or created within your physical system on this day.

XVI.   THERE IS ONLY CONSCIOUSNESS

Health, well-being, and all other desired outcomes have never been things you experience in some future moment or a result of some external factor. It is a state of mind you activate and actualize into your experience in your immediate Here and Now.

Health is an effect of consciousness, the state of being you keep yourself attuned to. Because you have so many contrary patterns of thought you have used to train yourself into experiences of dis-ease, you must cultivate the perspective of unfailing well-being. Let go of the rule sets that say "no-one can be healthy 100% of the time". Such conditions do not sever your ability to experience your reality the way you desire to experience it. The only rules there are, are the ones you have accepted without question. Be willing to question your rules for well-being.

Outward events cannot be the dictators of your experience and the beliefs and rules of others cannot be your standard for your quality of life.

Ask yourself, "what do I want to experience?"

If you are a being of Infinity, if what you are is an aspect of Infinite Intelligence, and if you right now exist in a field of Infinite Possibility, what kind of experiences do you and will you choose for yourself?

You must create and choose your own standards. Take responsibility for your state of being. Health is not something that happens to you. It is something you observe into being. You can choose your experience on all levels. Become your own authoritative source and release your philosophy of dis-ease. Acknowledge that your beliefs are not accidental or happenstance. The programs that form your world of experiences are not and were never random.

That you live in an energetic environment, that you have a network wiring of energy pathways in what you experience as your physical body, has only been invisible to you up to now because you have not given this reality much consideration and attention. Everything you experience as your world and physical body is a translation of a unique frequency field. There is nothing about your world; there is nothing in your world that is not energy.

You are a complex energetic system. Every layer of who you experience yourself to be is a unique configuration of wave-forms. And so, it is by changing the frequency of your being, the speed of vibration of your own consciousness, that you change the structure and appearance of your world. You do this by redefining not only your understanding of your world but of yourself as well. When you change the way you respond to your world, when you cease holding yourself to be at the mercy of outside forces, you allow yourself to experience your true power in this reality platform.

And that is what you are doing when you bring yourself to interact with a stream of consciousness, a flow of information, such as this one. Engage with these ideas consistently until you observe yourself responding to your world, your circumstances, differently. It is when these concepts are integrated into your consciousness matrix that you observe yourself behaving in a new way, from a new place within yourself.

The physical well-being you allow through the knowing of yourself as a field of consciousness in a vibrational environment will be invariable. When you hold your own state of being, your own consciousness, as the sole cause of all things in your world, your ability to know any potential outcome into being becomes un-wavering. You master not only your reality but your self as well. You master your ability to bring any outcome into visibility, into your experience for you become grounded in the understanding that consciousness is the sole cause and source of all, that there is no second cause or second author of your reality.

There is no "out there" to consult or resist. There is no outside force or factor to look to and plead with. You are not at the mercy of circumstances, conditions, labels, and appearances in the world of form. You are at cause. There is only consciousness, one's own power and ability to be, do, and have any experienced desired.

XVII.   YOUR POWER TO CHOOSE

There are no truths in this time-space reality that are unavailable to you. There are no definitions in this reality that you cannot expand, change, or dissolve. Every truth you hold as an unconditional truth is only a thought you have practiced and habituated. Every definition you have integrated into your outlook, into your consciousness-matrix, is subject to change. The reality you experience is entirely dependent upon the definitions, the rule-sets, you have imposed upon yourself. "Real" is only a matter of perception, of the perceptual boundaries you have set up for yourself. The lens through which you look through and experience your body-Universe reality is made up of a collection of truths, a web of beliefs, you have formed during your physical experience, and these web of beliefs can be altered by your own choice and focus. You are absolutely free to create and participate in the reality of your choosing. You are free to choose the vibrational density of the perception you utilize to experience your personal reality.

Every truth you hold is only a crystalized thought you are keeping active within your consciousness-matrix. And it is these crystalized forms of energy that you have formed in your physical focus that your body-Universe reality shapes itself around. The truths other's have created has nothing to do with you. The evidence of how other points of consciousness, other physical beings, have allowed or disallowed life energy has nothing to do with you. You can create your own evidence of well-being. You are the sole author of all that you make manifest in and as

your body-Universe reality.
You can create new truths and break free from the truths that no longer serve you. You can tune into the frequency domains that better serve the experiences of your preferred reality. As you find the vibration or frequency domain that feels good to you, you naturally open yourself up to the truths of that frequency domain, that simultaneous reality of well-being that has always been yours to experience. You choose consciously the realities you want to experience, for that is in your power.
You have endless, continuous, and constant access to pure energy. Every single one of your physical cells has countless energy channels, and your entire physical system is designed to be an energy conduit and a flawless energy flowing mechanism allowing you to experience the brilliance that is this time-space environment. Your body's own intelligence is pre-programmed to orchestrate everything necessary to be a thriving and balanced physical system. You are flawless and perfect in design at every level of your energetic structure and make-up, at every octave of your being, you are beyond all definition. What you are is boundlessness. What you are is an embodiment of complete freedom. What you are is an expression of infinite creativity. What you are is the miraculous power of the Universe itself.
The more you release the resistant patterns of thought you have accumulated, the more you move out of the flawed premise that resistance to absolute well-being is natural and normal, the more you experience your innate nature of absolute and unfailing well-being. Absolute well-being is the norm. Absolute and

unfailing well-being is the sole reality. Absolute unchanging wellness is the foundation of the forces that create worlds. And your alignment with this premise will make the power of your own being evident in your personal experience.

XVIII. DECLARATION OF POWER

Use the following declaration as a template to create your own. Take a moment each day to remind yourself that all the power of change and expansion is within yourself, it has always been within yourself.

Starting in this immediate instant, I cease allowing anything other than my own consciousness, my own choice of focus, to be the cause, the source, and authority of my physical experience. I now view the manifested world as it really is, as an outcome of my dominant vibration, my dominant patterns of thought and practiced web of beliefs. The world about me is only an effect of my own output, my own authorship. The world about can only indicate to me my own dominant vibrational signal, my chosen lens of perception. The world outside is only an mirroring to me my own self-image, who and what I know myself to be. I am at the root of everything I experience. I am the sole author of all that I make manifest in and as my physical reality.

There is nothing in my world that has appeared without my consent. I now recognize that I am the power in my own experience. I now know and recognize that everything is receiving its power from me, from my attention, focus, and acceptance of it as truth. I am the only one that can flow energy into beliefs and strengthen them. I am the only one who can accept and integrate programs into my personal matrix. I am the only one that can add power to my thoughts and beliefs. I am the only one that can set any thought into motion and power it until it manifests in my world. I am the only one that can agree to accept information as valid to my reality. And I am the only one that can withdraw my power of focus from the beliefs that don't serve me.

There is nothing in my view that is unchangeable. There is nothing in my view that is fixed, static, and determined. There is nothing in my world that is final. My reality is malleable. My world is a world of continual transformation and expansion. I now resolve to work with the cause of everything I experience. I now resolve to live in my power. I now resolve to choose and empower the reality I prefer to experience.

I am the sole author of all that I make manifest in and as my body-Universe reality.

You are the sole author of the body-Universe reality you materialize and participate in.

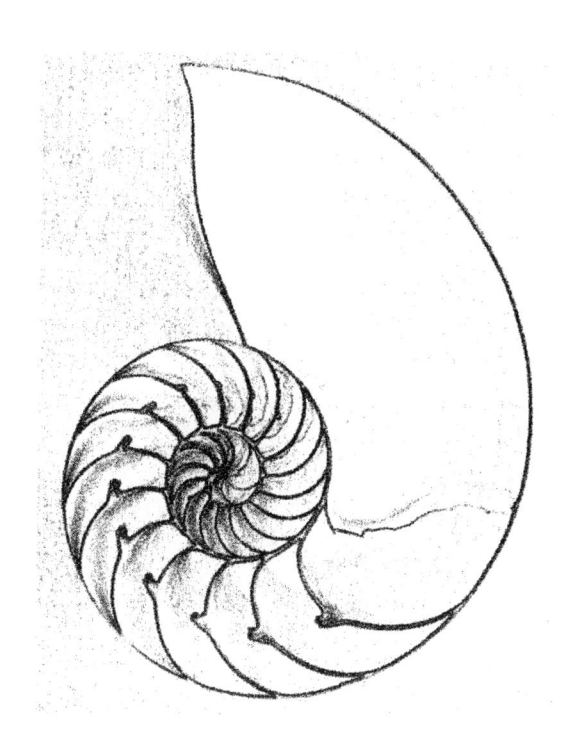

Acknowledgements

I am grateful for the teachings, pointers, and guidance that have opened my eyes and heart to the possibilities inherent within all beings. I acknowledge the many teachers in the world whose lives, whose work, and understanding are a constant invitation to wake up to the power within.

I am grateful for the texts and words of masters ancient and new who demonstrate and reflect the miraculous possibilities of this reality platform.

My deepest and heartfelt thanks to every being who has taken on and is taking on and will take on the work of awakening to the power, greatness, and potential within them.

I am grateful for my family and the friends who are constant sources of encouragement and support, and to the readers who have in their own consciousness contributed to the contents of my work.

Thank you for reading. Thank you for doing. Thank you for being.

Printed in Great Britain
by Amazon.co.uk, Ltd.,
Marston Gate.